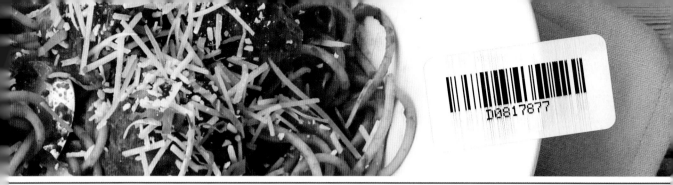

# without grain

## 100 Delicious Recipes for Eating a Grain-Free, Gluten-Free, Wheat-Free Diet

HAYLEY BARISA RYCZEK

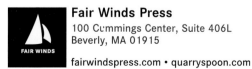

**Fair Winds Press**
100 Cummings Center, Suite 406L
Beverly, MA 01915

fairwindspress.com • quarryspoon.com

First published in the USA in 2015 by
Fair Winds Press, a member of
Quarto Publishing Group USA Inc.
100 Cummings Center
Suite 406-L
Beverly, MA 01915-6101
www.fairwindspress.com
Visit www.quarryspoon.com. It's your personal guide to a happy, healthy, and
extraordinary life!

19 18 17 16 15          2 3 4 5

ISBN: 978-1-59233-696-8

Digital edition published in 2015
eISBN: 978-1-62788-718-2

Library of Congress Cataloging-in-Publication Data available

Cover and book design by Carol Holtz
Page layout by Sporto
Photography by Hayley Barisa Ryczek
Printed and bound in China

*The information in this book is for educational purposes only. It is not intended
to replace the advice of a physician or medical practitioner. Please see your
health care provider before beginning any new health program.*

To my husband, Ray. I am grateful every day for having you in my life. Thank you for seeing in me what I fail to see in myself. It is your love and support that have made my dreams a reality.

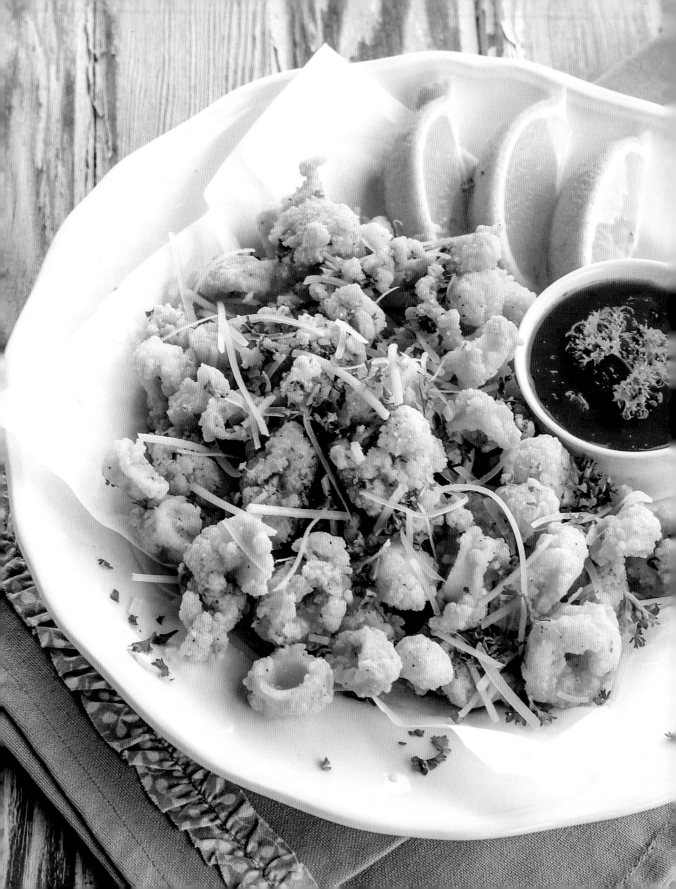

# CONTENTS

# INTRODUCTION

MY EARLIEST CHILDHOOD MEMORIES are of the weekends spent with my Grammie Elsie and Grandpa Stush. At the time, I enjoyed being with them because they spoiled me rotten. Looking back, however, I realize that I had no idea of the true abundance of gifts they were giving me. All those little intangibles (not the toys, clothes, and shoes) molded me into the person I am today.

Despite living in town with a small yard, my grandparents were known for their garden. I grew up eating freshly picked, still-dirty vegetables, while playing barefoot in their garden during the summer. And in the fall, I helped with putting up their harvest (canning, drying, and freezing).

As I grew older, Gram invited me to help with her catering business. You see, my grandmother was even more well known for her cooking! I learned to appreciate a well-made knife, how to season a cast-iron skillet, and the importance of adequately seasoning food, all under her tutelage.

After too long I was headed off to college, which took a toll on my body almost immediately. As my weight steadily climbed, it became apparent why I felt so awful. I was eating the standard collegiate diet of pizza, beer, sandwiches, soda, and French fries, which was vastly different from the real-foods diet I had eaten for the first eighteen years of my life.

Growing up, I ate homemade meals with my family, at the dinner table. My mom always served balanced meals with lots of vegetables and moderate amounts of protein. She didn't take shortcuts, such as using instant mashed potatoes or store-bought spaghetti sauce—after all, she learned to cook from my grandmother, too!

So, I ditched the cafeteria food and started cooking for myself. I never relied on recipes or cookbooks because cooking came naturally to me. I have always cooked just like my grandmother and my mother: with real foods, in their most natural state. I learned that when I ate balanced meals of real foods I felt healthy, but when I ate meals that were carbohydrate-heavy and full of processed foods, I felt awful.

Just as my passion for cooking grew, the trends in the 1990s pushed everyone toward a diet full of low-fat, processed foods. The idea of replacing natural foods with processed ones simply didn't make sense to me. I began researching health and saw beyond the low-fat fad and processed foods' "health" claims.

Over the subsequent fifteen-plus years, I continued researching healthy eating and finding ways to feel my best and maintain a healthy weight. I worked with alternative health professionals to help me understand why I wasn't able to easily lose weight and was increasingly struggling with my energy levels—even though I was eating a balanced diet of real foods, and I felt much better than if I had been eating the alternative.

After researching the effects of gluten, I removed it from my diet. Shortly afterward, genetic testing revealed I had received genes associated with both gluten intolerance and celiac disease. Celiac disease is a disorder that results in damage to the lining of the small intestine when foods containing gluten are eaten. Although I showed none of the classic symptoms (digestive upset, neurological issues, and mood disturbances), it became imperative that I remain gluten-free to avoid the damaging effects.

However, like so many people who've removed gluten from their diets, it wasn't enough for me to achieve optimal health. I noticed white patches of skin developing on the right side of my body, which quickly increased in number over a six-month period. Vitiligo is an autoimmune condition in which the skin loses its pigmentation (it's most commonly known as the skin condition Michael Jackson suffered from). With no known medical treatment or cure, many people find improvement by addressing their underlying inflammation (more on that in chapter 1).

By removing all grains from my diet, my vitiligo stopped spreading and many of my white patches began re-pigmenting. Seeing the immediate improvement in my condition ignited a passion in me for grain-free cooking and helping others improve their health as well.

I began blogging as a way to initially share my kitchen successes and homesteading experiences. (Not only did I inherit my grandmother's cooking notoriety but I also inherited her green thumb!) "Health Starts in the Kitchen" is my mantra for healthy living, and it's where I've been sharing my voice as a blogger. Today, www.healthstartsinthekitchen.com is known as one of the top web destinations for creative and delicious grain-free recipes.

In this book, you will find out how I live without grains, the reasons why I believe that grains are harming our bodies, why it's important to remove them from our diets, and which foods to replace them with. I'll also share with you 102 recipes for your favorite foods—such as fried chicken, soft pretzels, egg rolls, and pizza—all made *without grain*!

I'm excited to help you along your journey to health and wish you only the best.

In health,

*Hayley*

# Chapter 1:

# WHY GLUTEN-FREE ISN'T ENOUGH

ALTHOUGH GRAINS have become a diet staple, humans lived for more than 150,000 years without them as hunter-gatherers. We thrived on a scavenged diet of animals, nuts, seeds, leafy greens, tubers, and roots as well as seasonal fruits and vegetables. Around 10,000 years ago, with the advent of the agricultural revolution, our diet took a drastic change. As we settled down into communities and established towns, we began farming instead of foraging. The largest part of our diet that changed during that time was our consumption of grains. For the first time, we had the ability to grow, harvest, process, and prepare grains into an edible food on a regular basis. This process accelerated in the eighteenth and nineteenth centuries with the second agricultural revolution, which introduced new methods of farming that enabled grains to be cultivated on a large scale.

Today, the modern diet is awash in grains. They are touted as an inexpensive, easy-to-prepare, nutritious mainstay. Moreover, they are found in everything from the obvious (breads and cereals) to the not so obvious (salad dressings, condiments, and processed foods).

Although 10,000 years seems like a long time, it's actually a very short period of time as far as our evolutionary existence is concerned. Archaeological findings suggest that as grains became a regular part of our diet, we became a shorter and frailer species. The introduction of grains in the modern diet has also been strongly correlated with dramatically rising incidences of autoimmune illnesses, heart disease, diabetes, and cancer. Are grains the wonder food they are often touted to be by health experts on morning talk shows who extol the virtues of whole grain bread and "superfoods" such as oatmeal? Perhaps not.

The truth is that grain consumption, especially in the forms found today, is a major departure from the way humans have eaten for almost our entire evolutionary history. In the past 130 years of increased grain consumption, chronic disease rates have skyrocketed, fertility has fallen, and the average weight of the population has steadily risen.

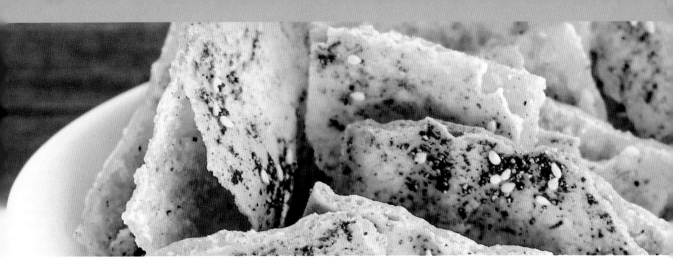

# HOW GRAINS AFFECT HEALTH

Grains can be problematic for many individuals, including those who do *not* have celiac disease or gluten sensitivity. Several aspects of eating grains can affect people in various ways.

## Lectins

Grains have a particularly high concentration of lectin, a class of plant proteins that evolved as a plant's way to naturally protect itself from insect predators. Lectins are typically concentrated in the plant's seeds, which are what we eat when we consume grains (and legumes, which also contain significant amounts of these lectins). The vegetables and fruits that we ate in large quantities before the introduction of grain into our diet are generally very low in lectins.

For some people, lectins can be hard to digest and can damage the cells that line the intestines—that is, the barrier between the intestines and the rest of the body—or cause spaces to open up between the gut cells. When this happens, these miniscule holes can allow particles of undigested food to leak out of the gut and into the bloodstream—otherwise known as leaky gut syndrome. This leaking is made worse by the fact that the lectins bind to sugars and other compounds in the gut that are then leaked into the bloodstream.

Your body thinks of these items as invaders and sets off an immune response, which shows up as inflammation. Chronic, low-grade inflammation is the precursor for many health conditions, including cardiovascular and autoimmune diseases. Leaky gut syndrome has also been connected to a variety of skin conditions, gastrointestinal problems, and mental disorders.

And, if damaging your gut lining and inflammation weren't enough, lectins can inhibit the absorption of many of the vitamins and minerals in your food. So even though you're eating an otherwise well-balanced diet, you are unable to use the vitamins and minerals you are ingesting.

## Acidic Foods

The indicator of a liquid's acidity or alkalinity is its pH value. Every liquid has a pH value that falls on a scale of 0 to 14, with 7 being neutral. A pH value lower than 7 is acidic; values greater than 7 indicate alkalinity. The adult body is about 60 percent fluid. This fluid fills every cell, the spaces between cells, and so forth. This fluid can be neutral, acidic, or alkaline. The body functions best when these fluids are neutral, which is to say neither acidic nor alkaline (7.0).

The body has natural mechanisms to eliminate acids. It can handle the natural acids created by the body in energy production and the process of rebuilding cells. However, the extra acidity created by a poor diet overwhelms the body's systems with a backlog of acids.

All food and drinks can be classified as alkaline, neutral, or acidic. Generally, meat, eggs, and fish are acidic, but we can balance them by eating lots of vegetables and some fruit, which are alkaline. Grains, however, are highly acidic foods. With such an abundance of grains in our diet, it is very challenging to eat enough alkaline foods to restore the balance, and the result is strain on the kidneys, liver, and pancreas.

## Omega-6 Fatty Acids

Fatty acids are called "essential" because our bodies can't produce them—we can only get them through the foods we eat. Both omega-3 and omega-6 fatty acids are important in all functions in our bodies, and their deficiencies have been linked to a host of problems, particularly those associated with heart health. Although both fatty acids are necessary, consuming too many omega-6s can crowd out the benefits of omega-3s.

Although the optimal ratio of omega-6 to omega-3 fats is 1:1, modern industrial societies such as ours consume anywhere between 20:1 and 60:1! Fatty fish (such as salmon), many vegetables, nuts, and flaxseed are typical sources of omega-3s. Grains, however, are high in linoleic acid, the omega-6 fatty acid that is linked to heart disease.

These omega-6 fatty acids are also highly concentrated in modern vegetable oils, which is how we end up ingesting more than we should. Oils derived from grains (and legumes), such as soy, safflower, sunflower, peanut, and corn, didn't exist until mechanical extraction was introduced into our food production. So we consume omega-6 fatty acids not only directly from grains, but also from the vegetable oils that we often cook them in. Talk about a double whammy!

Another way that omega-6s sneak into our bodies is through factory farm–raised meats. Cows, pigs, chickens, and farmed fish are fed grains. The meat produced from these animals no longer contains a healthy 1:1 ratio of omega-6 to omega-3 fatty acids. Instead, it is typically closer to 10:1. It is not enough just to avoid grains in your diet; you need to be mindful of what you eat that eats grains too and make a concerted effort to consume pasture-raised animals and wild-caught fish.

# GLUTEN CROSS-REACTIVITY

For many people who avoid gluten because of celiac disease or gluten intolerance, a gluten-free diet isn't enough because although they may feel some improvement, they continue to experience symptoms. According to a 2009 study of celiac disease patients in *The Journal of Alimentary Pharmacology and Therapeutics*, only 8 percent of those participating in the study reached "histological normalization" after following a strict gluten-free diet for sixteen months, meaning that their gut tissue completely recovered to that of a healthy person. This leaves 92 percent who continued to suffer with symptoms.

Sometimes the continuing symptoms are the result of gluten cross-contamination—i.e., something thought to be gluten-free came in contact with gluten. This often happens when consuming food in restaurants where gluten-containing and gluten-free foods are prepared in the same space or when typically gluten-free foods (such as oats) are processed at facilities that also process gluten-containing foods. Continuing symptoms may also indicate that the body simply requires more time to fully heal from a lifetime of gluten consumption. However, it may not be either of these reasons. Instead, the culprit might be gluten cross-reactivity.

Gluten cross-reactivity is an immune reaction in which gluten antibodies react with the proteins in other foods, such as gluten-free grains. Even though these foods don't contain gluten, the body reacts as if they do. Proteins are made of long chains of amino acids. The specific sequence of these amino acids—how the links of the chain are put together—is what determines what kind of protein it is. For example, antibodies are proteins produced by immune cells that identify and help remove invaders in the body. There are five types of antibodies, each with distinctive functions within the body, but to keep things simple, we're going to touch on the three types relevant to the foods we eat.

**IgE antibodies** are responsible for allergic reactions, such as when someone goes into anaphylaxis after eating nuts.

**IgG** and **IgA antibodies** are critical for protecting us from pathogens (disease, illness, and so on) but are also responsible for reactions to food sensitivities and intolerances. Both IgG and IgA antibodies are secreted by our immune cells into the lymphatic system, bodily fluids, and tissues. And because many IgG and IgA antibodies are found in the tissues and fluids surrounding the gut, our gut is considered one of the main components of our immune system.

When antibodies are created in reaction to a protein, they are programmed to recognize a small sequence of amino acids within that protein. Because the antibody is created in response to only a small section of an amino acid rather than the entire amino acid, often many different antibodies will form against the same food. This is part of the reason certain foods have a higher potential to cause allergic responses and sensitivities.

The same amino acid sequence that antibodies react to in gluten is also present in other proteins from different foods. Though there are only twenty-one different amino acids, there are millions of possible ways a group of amino acids can be put together to form a protein; however, similar amino acid sequences are often repeated in many non–gluten containing foods.

To avoid all gluten and cross-reactive grains, it's advisable to avoid *all* of the following foods:

- Wheat (white, whole, graham, pastry, etc.)
- Durum
- Semolina
- Einkorn
- Spelt
- Kamut
- Farro/emmer
- Bulgur
- Barley (malt)
- Rye
- Triticale
- Wheat berries
- Oats
- Sorghum
- Millet
- Teff
- Corn (maize)
- Rice (including brown, not wild*)
- Amaranth**
- Buckwheat**
- Quinoa**

*Wild rice is not directly related to Asian rice, although they are close cousins. There are no reported cross-reactivity issues with wild rice, but be sure to confirm wild rice is the only ingredient and that there was no risk of cross-contamination during processing.*

** *These "pseudo" grains are actually seeds that are high in glutamic acid and should be avoided in addition to all other true cereal grains.*

In addition to grains and pseudo grains, there are other foods that are known to cause an antibody reaction in the body. If, after removing the previous list of foods from your diet, you are still experiencing symptoms, consider removing these additional foods from your diet and see whether your symptoms improve:

- Potatoes
- Soy
- Dairy
- Chocolate
- Yeast
- Coffee (instant)
- Sesame
- Tapioca (cassava or yucca)
- Eggs

Although many recipes in this book include these potentially problematic foods, I have included a section on allergy-free substitutions on page 198 with suggestions for recipe modifications. No recipes in this book contain soy or coffee.

## WHO SHOULD AVOID GRAINS?

Every day more people are diagnosed with celiac disease and even more with gluten sensitivity. For these people, a grain-free diet is absolutely essential. However, there are even more people needlessly suffering from disease and illness often related to an antibody response to the foods they eat.

There are more than 100 confirmed autoimmune diseases—for example, celiac disease, multiple sclerosis, rheumatoid arthritis, type 1 diabetes—and many more that are suspected of being autoimmune related. Although the symptoms vary significantly, the root cause of all these diseases remains the same: our immune system is attacking our own cells. With autoimmune diseases, something causes the body to attack itself. Removing grains from your diet is a good step in strengthening your immune system.

There are also several other ailments that are known to occur frequently in conjunction with autoimmune diseases that can benefit from a grain-free diet:

- Cholangitis
- Chronic fatigue syndrome
- Eczema
- Fibromyalgia
- Polycystic ovary syndrome (PCOS)

Additionally, if you have any of the following symptoms, many of which are linked to undiagnosed autoimmune conditions and/or food allergies or intolerances, a grain-free diet may be beneficial:

- Allergies
- Anxiety
- Blood pressure changes (typically low)
- Depression
- Digestive issues
- Fatigue
- Frequent illness and infections
- Gallbladder disease
- Low blood sugar
- Malaise (an overall feeling of being unwell)
- Memory issues
- Migraines and recurrent headaches
- Muscle or joint pain
- Muscle weakness
- PMS
- Rashes and other skin problems
- Resistance to weight loss
- Sleep disturbances
- Swollen glands
- Thyroid issues
- Yeast infections

## THE HEALTHY GRAIN MYTH

As we've just seen, grains are not the wonder food they are often touted to be. They can damage the gut lining, cause inflammation, and contribute to an overly acidic body. Going grain-free is not only beneficial to those with celiac disease and gluten intolerance, but doing so may benefit many people with various other conditions and autoimmune diseases as well. But how can eliminating grains be beneficial to so many people, when we are constantly told that grains (and lots of them) are an essential part of a healthy diet?

Despite what we are led to believe by whole grain–promoting television commercials and food product labels, grains aren't the nutritional powerhouses they are advertised to be. Although grains can be a source of essential vitamins and minerals such as $B_1$, $B_2$, magnesium, iron, zinc, and potassium, there are more effective ways to get these nutrients into your diet—without a high-glycemic, carbohydrate-rich, bulky grain. A serving of so-called "healthy whole grains" isn't as nutritionally dense as a colorful salad or plate full of vegetables! Doesn't it make more sense to get your nutrients from eating a variety of vegetables, fruits, proteins, and healthy fats? Not only do they offer higher nutrient profiles, but they also don't come with the potential drawbacks associated with eating grains.

## WHAT ABOUT FIBER?

One of the first questions people ask me when I suggest they try out a grain-free diet is, "What about fiber?" Fiber is an important part of a healthy diet, but grains are not its only source. You will have no problem getting enough fiber from fruits and vegetables; avocadoes, broccoli, sweet potatoes, artichokes, spinach, and carrots are all excellent sources.

If you are specifically worried about staying "regular," the secret to a healthy digestive system is not eating more whole-grain fiber, it's keeping adequate levels of good bacteria in your gut. The natural bacteria in your large intestine helps make up stool bulk, maintain water content to ease digestion and constipation, and soften the stool. Fiber, particularly excessive insoluble fiber found in grains, can offer a quick jump-start to get things moving, but it is not the natural catalyst for keeping your digestive system running smoothly. Eliminating grains that may have damaged your gut is an essential first step to creating an environment in which good bacteria will multiply. It's also very important to replenish the good bacteria in your gut by incorporating fermented foods and drinks into your grain-free diet.

## STAY REGULAR WITH FERMENTED FOODS NOT GRAINS

Before modern refrigeration, people sought other methods to preserve food and mitigate spoilage. Using naturally occurring bacteria and yeast to ferment native foodstuffs didn't only protect food from spoilage, but it also added probiotic foods to their diet and boosted their nutritional intake. Not only that, but many fermented foods contain enzymes that humans need to more effectively obtain nutrition from their food. Whether they knew it or not, ancient peoples benefited in many ways from fermented foods. Adding fermented foods to your diet is an inexpensive and delicious way to speed your body's healing process and help eliminate your symptoms.

**Fermented foods improve digestion.**
Fermenting our foods before we eat them is akin to partially digesting them first. According to Joanne Slavin, PhD, RD, a professor in the Department of Food Science and Nutrition at the University of Minnesota, "Sometimes people who cannot tolerate milk can eat yogurt. That's because the lactose [which is usually the part people can't tolerate] in milk is broken down as the milk is fermented and turns into yogurt." Getting the good bacteria working makes the job easier on our guts.

**Fermented foods restore the proper balance of bacteria in the gut.** Do you suffer from lactose intolerance? Gluten intolerance? Constipation? Irritable bowel syndrome? Yeast infections? Allergies? Asthma? All of these conditions have been linked to a lack of good bacteria in the gut.

**Fermented foods are rich in enzymes.**
Your body needs enzymes to adequately digest, absorb, and utilize the nutrients in your food. As we age, our body's supply of enzymes goes down, making it increasingly important to add them via our food.

**Fermenting food increases its vitamin content.** Fermented dairy products show an increased level of folic acid, which is critical to producing healthy babies, as well as pyridoxine, B vitamins, riboflavin, and biotin, depending on the strains of bacteria present.

**Fermented food helps with nutrient absorption.** You can ingest huge amounts of nutrients, but unless your body actually *absorbs* them, they're useless to you. When you improve digestion, you improve absorption.

### INCORPORATING FERMENTED FOODS INTO YOUR DIET

Start by switching from pasteurized, vinegar-brined condiments to the live, fermented versions of pickles, sauerkraut, salsa, ketchup, sour cream, kimchi, and yogurt. You can also drink 2 to 3 ounces (60 to 90 ml) of fermented beverages every couple of days. Kombucha, kvass, and unpasteurized kefir are readily available at many health food stores.

## TAKE THE 90-DAY CHALLENGE

I encourage you to go without grain for at least 90 days to give your body ample time to adjust to your new way of eating. You have nothing to lose (but poor health), and you can always go back to eating grains. This is your opportunity to start down a healthier path and take a proactive approach to healing your body. (Obviously, it's always prudent to run any major dietary changes past a licensed health care practitioner.)

At the end of 90 days, you will most likely notice that you feel better than you can remember. Digestive issues such as gas and a bloated tummy probably will have abated. You might see improved energy levels and sharper thinking. Maybe you'll even lose a few pounds because you cut empty carbohydrates out of your diet! Most important, you won't have any more desire to eat grains because you'll have an understanding of how they have negatively affected your health.

I know it's a big step, but there's no need to worry! I'm going to make the transition to a grain-free diet very easy. The rest of this book is dedicated to helping guide you every step of the way. Let's get started!

# Chapter 2:

# HOW TO GO GRAIN-FREE: WHAT TO EAT AND WHAT TO AVOID

I COMPLETELY UNDERSTAND how overwhelming it can seem to go grain-free, but don't worry—you'll catch on quickly.

Eating grain-free isn't complicated when you stay away from packaged and processed foods. It's a no-brainer that foods such as steak, chicken thighs, broccoli, sweet potatoes, and apples are all grain-free, unlike packaged foods with long lists of ingredients, such as crackers, cereals, and granola bars.

Unfortunately, there is no such thing as a comprehensive list of all food items that contain grains. Manufacturers regularly change their ingredients, mislabel, have product recalls, and so on. This is why my best advice is to avoid processed and packaged foods as much as possible. It's also a good idea to prepare your own meals at home, where you can control what goes into your food, instead of eating out. (See page 197 for my tips on eating out without grains.)

## COMMON SOURCES OF HIDDEN GRAINS

Grains are sneaky, and you may be surprised at all the places they hide! I've pulled together this section that lists the most common foods to avoid as well as other items and additives that you should be cautious of. As you can see from the categories that follow, in addition to the list of grains and cross-reactive grains on page 12, you're better off sticking with real foods and ditching the processed, packaged stuff. There's no way grains can sneak into fresh broccoli, right?

### Alcoholic Beverages

The most important thing to remember when having a cocktail is don't drink the wrong ones. If you're going to imbibe, stick to wine (not wine coolers), champagne, tequila, rum, or vodka made from potatoes or fruit. Avoid grain-based spirits (gin, whiskey, scotch, rye, bourbon, or moonshine vodka), malted beverages (hard iced teas and lemonades), schnapps (often a blend of liquors made from fruit and liquors made from grains), and beer.

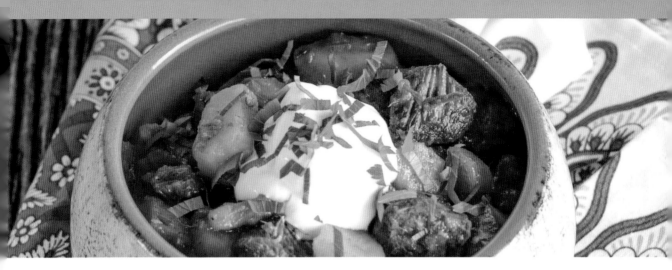

It should be noted that manufacturers often consider their distilled alcoholic spirits (hard liquors) to be gluten- and grain-free; they claim that distillation eliminates any traces of gluten or grains. However, because many people still react to these spirits, I strongly recommend against the consumption of any beverage derived from grain regardless of manufacturer claims. It's better to be safe than sorry.

## Nonedible Items

One often overlooked area for grain and gluten ingredients is the products we use—those that come into contact with our skin or those we ingest, but aren't specifically foods. Something as innocent as taking Communion wafers, licking a stamp, or applying lotions can prevent the most sensitive of people from fully healing. Keep in mind that our skin is the largest organ of our body, and what it absorbs can affect our health. To ensure you are not accidentally contaminating yourself, read product labels; look for allergy statements that products are gluten-free and not processed in a facility that could cause cross-contamination. When in doubt, do without.

Potentially allergenic products include the following:

- Stamps and envelopes
- Toothpaste
- Makeup and lipstick
- Shampoo, conditioner, and hair-styling products
- Detergents and soaps
- Medications
- Vitamin supplements
- Lotions
- Play dough

## Food Additives and Processed Foods

Not only are processed foods dangerous to your health (because of the processing itself), but also they often harbor hidden sources of grains in ingredients and additives. If you choose to eat processed foods, carefully read the ingredient labels to avoid any chance of consuming grains. It's a good idea to also check with the manufacturers when in doubt. See the chart on page 18 for a list of food additives and processed foods to either avoid or treat with caution because they may contain grains.

# COMMON ADDITIVES AND PROCESSED FOODS
# THAT MAY CONTAIN GRAIN

Monosodium glutamate (MSG)

Modified food starch

Textured vegetable protein (TVP)
and vegetable protein

Hydrolyzed plant protein

Hydrolyzed vegetable protein

Hydrogenated starch hydrolysate

Hydroxypropylated starch

Pregelatinized starch

Vegetable gums (guar and xanthan gums)

Extenders and binders

Maltodextrin (wheat- or corn-based)

Dextrin

Maltose (malt sugar)

Seasonings

Natural flavors

Smoke flavors

Artificial flavors

Natural colors

Artificial colors

Caramel color and flavoring

Soy sauce and tamari (Coconut aminos
is an excellent replacement.)

Miso

Bouillon cubes or stock cubes (Learn to
make your own bone broth on page 93
instead.)

Chicken stock

Candy (It may be dusted with wheat flour.)

Canned soups

Cheese spreads and other processed
cheese foods

Chocolate (It may contain malt flavoring.)

Cold cuts, wieners, and sausages (They may
have gluten from cereal fillers.)

Dip mixes

Dry sauce mixes

Honey hams (They may contain gluten in
the coating.)

Ice cream and frozen yogurt

Instant coffee and iced tea

Malt vinegar and distilled white vinegar

Corn oil

Precooked/seasoned poultry and meats
(Verify that the flavorings and seasoning are
grain-free.)

Sour cream (It may contain modified food
starch of indeterminate source.)

Dry-roasted and honey-roasted nuts

Fried foods (The same oil may be used for
wheat-containing items.)

Gravies (Check out the thickening agent and
liquid base.)

Baking powder (It commonly contains wheat
or corn; see recipe, page 20.)

# STOCKING A GRAIN-FREE PANTRY

Keeping a well-stocked, grain-free kitchen is essential for sticking to a healthy lifestyle. If you have healthy foods at your fingertips and no processed foods to fall back on, then you won't be tempted to reach for the cereal box on a busy morning.

The best way to make the switch is to do a complete kitchen overhaul. If you still have those grain-containing foods in the fridge or cupboard, I promise that eventually you'll either give in to temptation or, worse, sabotage your health by accidentally eating grains!

## Guide to Grain-Free Flours and Starches

One of the biggest obstacles to overcome with grain-free cooking is how to substitute grain-free flours and starches in place of all-purpose flour in your favorite recipes. Though there's no one formula that will work in every case, once you've become familiar with the properties of the different grain-free flours and find awesome recipes that put them together (such as those in this book), you'll be back to enjoying all your favorite foods in no time.

### MOST COMMON SUBSTITUTES

Although there is a wide variety of grain-free flours available, I use these the most often with the best results.

**Blanched almond flour** is the most popular grain-free flour substitute. It is made of finely ground almonds that have been blanched and their skins removed. A high-quality blanched almond flour (such as Honeyville Farms) is very finely milled and can be quite light compared to other nut and seed flours. Generally, it measures 1:1 when substituting for wheat flour. It works well in baking when you want a denser crumb, such as in muffins, coffee cakes, and chewy cookies. In recipes that have a large amount of wet ingredients, adding starch or coconut flour can be helpful. Note: Do not use almond meal in place of blanched almond flour because it is too coarse. Substitutions for blanched almond flour include sunflower seed flour (which tends to turn a bit greenish when used with baking soda but is not unsafe to eat), hazelnut flour, and chestnut flour (which is slightly sweeter).

**Coconut flour** has a high fiber content and absorbs liquid efficiently. It is a tricky flour to work with; often 1 teaspoon can make the difference between the texture you are going for and something completely different. When you add coconut flour to wet ingredients, the batter will thicken as it sits, which isn't a bad thing, before putting it in the oven. The general rule of thumb is to replace one-fourth of the wheat flour with coconut flour.

**Arrowroot starch** (also known as arrowroot powder) is dehydrated and ground arrowroot tuber. It is mostly a starch and is great for adding lightness to a recipe, as well as for thickening sauces without a roux. Arrowroot starch can replace cornstarch in recipes 1:1. If replacing wheat flour with arrowroot starch to add

## Homemade Grain-Free Baking Powder

When on a grain-free diet, avoid commercial baking powder because cornstarch is the main ingredient. Also, with more than 80 percent of corn in the United States now genetically modified (GM or GMO), making your own baking powder will help eliminate another sneaky source of GMOs in your home.

**1 cup (72 g) cream of tartar**
**½ cup (110 g) baking soda**
**½ cup (64 g) arrowroot starch**

Mix the cream of tartar, baking soda, and arrowroot starch together and store in an airtight container. Use in place of commercial baking powder in recipes.

### Yield: Approximately 2 cups (240 g)

lightness to a recipe, substitute up to one-fourth of your flour with arrowroot.

**Tapioca starch** comes from the ground cassava (also known as yucca, yuca, manioc, or tapioca) root. This is not the same as arrowroot powder. Even though people use tapioca and arrowroot interchangeably, they have different properties in baking. Tapioca adds elasticity to baking, helping to bind and give more bounce. It isn't a good substitute for thickening sauces and gravies, however, because it gets stringy and gluey. You can replace up to about half of the flour normally called for in a recipe with tapioca starch.

**Potato starch** is often used as a thickener for sauces, soups, and stews. Potato starch tolerates higher temperatures better than cornstarch when used as a thickener. It's a natural way to add moistness to many baked goods.

**Potato flour** is a powder made from ground potatoes that is commonly used in baking. Some cooks use it as a thickener, and it can also add flavor and texture to foods such as cakes, breads, and cookies. Jewish cooks sometimes also use it when preparing foods according to Passover dietary restrictions, which prohibit the use of many grains. Potato flour is often confused with the similar-sounding potato *starch* flour, but they are not to be used interchangeably.

### WHICH FLOURS AND STARCHES TO USE

When you first give up grains, you'll notice how difficult it can be to find the treats you used to enjoy. Premade and packaged goods bearing labels that appear to be healthy are usually anything but, thanks to the additives and ingredients they use. Baking at home with grain-free flours and healthier, real-food ingredients gives you the satisfaction of an occasional treat without the inflammatory ingredients.

Before you attempt to bake or cook without grains, it's helpful to understand what role grains, and more specifically gluten, play in various recipes.

Wheat flour (more commonly known as all-purpose flour) is the main ingredient in everything from pasta or pizza dough to cakes and cookies. There are two main proteins in wheat flour: glutenin and gliadin. Glutenin provides most of the strength and elasticity in dough, allowing it to bounce back after being stretched. Gliadin, on the other hand, provides the actual stretching.

When you remove wheat flour from your favorite recipes, consider the role the flour plays in the recipe so that you can devise a successful plan for substitution.

**Thickener:** In sauces, gravies, soups, and stews, wheat flour and cornstarch most often play the role of thickener. When the starch granules are heated, they absorb water and form a gelatinous network, which is how a few tablespoons (24 to 32 g) of flour can turn chicken stock into gravy. It's easy to replace flour with a grain-free alternative thickener, such as arrowroot and potato starch, using a 1:1 ratio.

**Coating and Breading:** Flour is also used as a coating in dishes such as fried chicken or breaded pork chops. The starches in the flour are responsible for browning and crisping, while the

protein in the flour helps the flour coat and cling to the surface of the food. Using a combination of grain-free flours that mix starch and protein will produce the best results, as in my Breading Mix (page 34), where I use a combination of starches (arrowroot and tapioca) with blanched almond flour (protein).

**Structure in Baked Goods:** The main use for flour in the home kitchen is to give structure to baked goods. This is where gluten performs the essential function of expanding proteins to trap gas bubbles; it is key to the texture of many baked goods. While it's not difficult to find substitutions for thickeners and coatings that are grain-free, replicating these structural properties is much more challenging.

Wheat flour in baked goods has a starch content of approximately 75 percent; however, most often with grain-free substitutions, you will have even more starch content. Less protein means batters and doughs can't hold the air bubbles as well, and the end result can be heavier and denser. Many times, grain-free recipe adaptations can benefit from additional baking powder (page 20), baking soda, or yeast. Both baking powder and baking soda are chemical leavening agents that cause batters to rise when baked; baking soda requires the addition of an acidic ingredient, such as vinegar, citrus juice, sour cream, yogurt, buttermilk, chocolate, cocoa (not Dutch-processed), honey, molasses (also brown sugar), fruits, or maple syrup.

## Beware the Additives

Many packaged gluten-free products and recipes (though none in this book) use additives to help replicate the properties of gluten. The two most common additives are xanthan gum and guar gum, and both need to be avoided.

XANTHAN GUM is the result of mixing corn sugar and bacteria called *Xanthomonas campestris*. It is used as both a thickening agent and replacement for gluten in many recipes. It's also notorious for causing digestive upset in sensitive individuals. A xanthan reaction may include migraine headaches, skin itchiness, and—if exposed to large amounts, such as bakery workers are—nose and throat irritation.

GUAR GUM is much like xanthan gum except that it is actually an extract from the guar plant. Their usage is very nearly the same. Guar gum combines with water molecules to form a gel-like substance. Until 1990, it was used as one of the main ingredients in many nonprescription diet pills for its "fullness" effect. The FDA banned its use in such pills when claims arose linking it to many digestive issues.

One of the keys to successful grain-free baking is letting go of your expectations of what batters and dough "should" be. Because of the high starch content of grain-free flours, adding more liquid is often necessary for proper hydration. For example, when you make Sliceable Sandwich Bread (pages 38 to 39), the dough will seem too wet in comparison to its wheat flour counterpart.

When measuring grain-free flours by the cup, use the "dip and sweep method" unless a different method of measurement is specified. To do this, dip the measuring cup into the container of flour and level it off by drawing a butter knife (or other flat-edged utensil) over the top of the measuring cup. Pouring or dumping the flour into the measuring cup will most often result in less flour making it into the recipe than what is needed.

When first attempting to convert a recipe, the classic grain-free substitution is blanched almond flour on its own or in conjunction with arrowroot starch, tapioca starch, and/or coconut flour. These ingredients are easy to find, and they behave predictably in recipes. Whenever I am creating a grain-free version of a traditional recipe, I start out using my basic grain-free flour blend (equal parts blanched almond flour, arrowroot starch, and tapioca starch) to replace the flour, and I anticipate needing to increase the amount by at least 25 percent (e.g., 1 cup [125 g] all-purpose flour = 1¼ cups [150 g] grain-free flour blend) because the grain-free blend is not as absorptive. After years of experimenting, I've learned how to gauge the moisture in doughs and batters to determine whether I need any additional liquids. And if I do need to add liquids, it's best to extend the baking time a little to help dry out baked goods, especially breads. With experience and practice, you'll be adapting and creating your own grain-free recipes as well. See page 199 for the brands of grain-free flours and starches I use and recommend.

## Fats and Oils

You'll notice that I frequently refer to cooking fats in the following recipes. Fat—provided it is the right kind of fat—can play an important nutritional role in grain-free eating. If you are new to grain-free eating, you are probably used to getting sated on grain-laden carbs. Fat takes longer to digest so it will help you feel fuller longer. Moreover, if you are trying to heal a damaged gut brought on by years of consuming allergy-provoking grains, fat can provide an important role in helping soothe inflammation and repair leaky gut syndrome. In addition to helping you feel fuller longer, balancing your blood sugar, and providing vital nutrients, good fats also provide a patch and repair function on damaged intestinal lining.

Learning about fats can be confusing. It seems that wherever we turn, we're confronted with advertisements and "experts" telling us that low-fat, reduced-fat, or fat-free products are healthier for us, which in fact couldn't be further from the truth.

Fat is an essential nutrient that we cannot live without. The human brain is approximately 60 percent fat, and fat plays a key role in the nervous system; hormone production and regulation; smoother, younger-looking skin; and every cell in the body. Dietary fat delivers omega-3 and omega-6 fatty acids as well fat-soluble vitamins A, D, E, and K throughout our bodies. Fat is also how the body stores extra energy so that in times of famine, the body can draw on its fat stores for survival. It's a vital component of breast milk, and fat is the single most important factor in an infant's optimal brain development.

When it comes to the fats that you should (or shouldn't) be eating, I've grouped them into three categories—cooking fats, cold fats, and toxic fats—to make it a little easier to understand.

### COOKING FATS

Saturated fats are the best options for cooking because they are chemically stable and resistant to damage from heat. Always choose fats from organic and/or grass-fed sources. In my recipes, you'll notice that I frequently call for a general "cooking fat"; in those instances, feel free to use whichever of these fats you prefer. However, in places where I call for a specific fat (such as butter in my Pie Crust, page 33), use what is recommended for the best results.

Use these oils for cooking, baking, frying, and sautéing:

- Butter, ghee, and clarified butter
- Lard (rendered pork fat) or reserved bacon drippings
- Tallow (rendered beef fat)
- Schmaltz (rendered poultry fat)
- Coconut oil and unrefined, virgin coconut oil
- Palm oil and red palm oil

## COLD FATS

These fats and oils are a healthy addition to your diet. They are best organic and should be unrefined and expeller or cold pressed to avoid the high heat and chemical processing that can damage them. And just as high heat from processing can damage these oils, it's best to use these fats for salads, sauces, or condiments where they will not be heated to retain the most health benefits:

- Olive oil
- Avocado oil
- Macadamia nut oil
- Walnut oil
- Sesame oil

## TOXIC FATS

These fats are highly processed, easily damaged, or synthetic. They oxidize easily and become rancid, causing inflammation in the body. According to Mary Enig, in *Know Your Fats*, oxidized, or rancid, oils enter the body and are recognized not as food, but as toxins. Our body does not metabolize toxins but instead stores them in our fat cells, which leads to inflammation. These fats also have a high polyunsaturated fatty acid (PUFA) content, and they are too high in omega-6 fatty acids (see the dangers of too much omega-6s on page 10). This category includes any fat that is hydrogenated or partially hydrogenated:

- Margarine, oleo, or other butter substitutes
- Vegetable oil
- Soybean oil
- Canola oil
- Corn oil
- Cottonseed oil
- Safflower oil
- Sunflower oil
- Rice bran oil
- Grapeseed oil
- Vegetable shortening

## JUST SAY "NO" TO PROCESSED FOOD

Resisting the urge to drink that soda or eat those chips can be tough, especially if you have grown accustomed to eating these highly addictive foods as part of your diet. But once you understand how these and other processed foods affect your mind and body, it becomes easier to make healthier food choices that enrich your health rather than deplete it.

Fresh foods are actually cheaper than processed foods. People with junk food addictions often claim that fresh, healthy foods are too expensive. But according to numerous studies and assessments, meals and snacks made from scratch end up costing less per serving than their unhealthy, processed equivalents. For example, a single serving of chili made with fresh, organic ingredients and grass-fed beef is about 50 cents cheaper to make than buying an individual bowl of chemical-laden, microwaveable chili from the grocery store. And keep in mind how sneakily grains can find their way into those packaged and processed foods (see page 18), in addition to the following ways they are damaging to your health.

**Processed foods are highly addictive.** Your body processes whole foods much differently than it does refined, processed, and heavily modified "junk" foods. Processed foods tend to overstimulate the production of dopamine, also known as the "pleasure" neurotransmitter, which makes you crave them constantly. Your body ends up not being able to resist the temptation to continue eating junk foods in excess, which can lead to obesity and other health problems.

**Processed foods often contain phosphates.** These could wreak havoc on your organs and bones. These phosphate additives augment taste, texture, and shelf life, but they are also associated with health problems, such as rapid aging, kidney deterioration, and weak bones.

**Processed food consumption is linked to chronic inflammation.** One of the leading causes of chronic illness today is inflammation. And studies continue to show that refined sugars, processed grains, vegetable oils, and many other ingredients commonly found in processed foods are associated with this inflammation epidemic. So, the next time you crave a candy bar or a box of cheese crackers and you're ready to give in, consider that heart disease, dementia, neurological problems, respiratory failure, and cancer have all been linked to the chronic inflammation caused by processed food consumption.

**Processed foods can disrupt digestion.** Because they have been stripped of their natural fibers, enzymes, vitamins, and other nutrients, processed foods tend to wreak havoc on the digestive tract. Chronic consumption of such foods can throw your internal ecosystem off balance, harming beneficial bacteria, feeding harmful bacteria, and exposing your system to disease and illness.

**Processed foods can affect your mood.** If you suffer from chronic bouts of "brain fog" or have difficulty concentrating and thinking normally, chances are your diet has something to do with it. A 2013 study out of Oxford University found that junk food consumption can cause people to become angry and irritable. Nutrient-dense whole foods, on the other hand, can help level out your mood, sustain your energy levels, and leave you feeling calmer and more focused.

**Processed foods are loaded with GMOs.** The basic buildings blocks of most processed foods on the market today are derived from laboratories, not nature. A GMO (genetically modified organism) is the result of the laboratory process of taking genes from one species and inserting them into another in an attempt to obtain a desired trait or characteristic; hence, they are also known as transgenic organisms. This process may be called either genetic engineering (GE) or genetic modification (GM); they are one and the same.

The American Academy of Environmental Medicine (AAEM) reported that "several animal studies indicate serious health risks associated with GMOs," including infertility, immune problems, accelerated aging, faulty insulin regulation, and changes in major organs and the gastrointestinal system. The AAEM asked physicians to advise patients to avoid GM foods.

A number of studies over the past decade have revealed that genetically engineered foods can pose serious risks to farmers, human health, domesticated animals, wildlife, and the environment, yet GMOs are now present in 75 to 80 percent of conventional processed food in the United States, according to the Grocery Manufacturers Association.

## Common GMO Crops

Currently commercialized GM crops in the United States include soy (94 percent), cotton (90 percent), canola (90 percent), sugar beets (95 percent), corn (88 percent), Hawaiian papaya (more than 50 percent), and zucchini and yellow squash (more than 24,000 acres). Although wheat is not a genetically modified organism (GMO), evidence suggests that GM foods, such as soy and corn, may help explain the recent explosion of gluten-related disorders, which now affect up to 18 million Americans.

**Processed foods are loaded with pesticides.** To effectively grow the foods that are then processed into grocery store merchandise, conventional farmers apply pesticides and herbicides, many of which end up in the final product they are growing. Breakfast cereals alone have been found to contain up to seventy different types of pesticides, including warehouse fumigation chemicals and other residues.

**Processed foods are not actually food.** One of the ways you can assess the nutritional value of food is to see how animals, insects, bacteria, and fungi respond to it. Real foods will actually rot or grow mold, for instance, while fake, processed foods remain largely the same in appearance and shape no matter what their age. If these foods don't mold or rot outside of the body, how can we assume that our bodies can properly digest and use nutrients from them?

### Going Organic

No matter where you live, you have to deal with pollution: in the air you breathe, in the water you drink, and in the foods you eat. You can do little about air pollution, but you can filter the water you drink, and you can choose to consume organic food. The pollution in our food comes in several different forms:

- Pesticides: insecticides, herbicides, and fungicides
- Food additives: preservatives, artificial colors, flavor enhancers, etc.

- GMOs: a gene from one organism is spliced into another organism to develop a specific trait that does not otherwise exist naturally
- Artificial hormones and antibiotics to speed the growth of livestock or production of milk

Many pesticide residues can remain on conventionally raised vegetables and fruits even after washing. Some studies have discovered the residue of as many as thirty-seven different pesticides on the skins of conventionally grown apples. Peeling fruits and vegetables removes the residues—but also many of the nutrients that are found in or just under the skins. Young children are especially susceptible to pesticide residues because their bodies are still developing, and they tend to consume proportionally more fruit per pound than adults. Organic fruits and vegetables are produced without synthetic chemicals, although organic pesticides are sometimes used.

Organically raised cattle are allowed access outside to graze on grass, are fed organically grown feed, are not given artificial hormones to speed their growth or their production of milk, and are not given antibiotics as a disease preventive. Chickens and pigs are given organically grown feed, allowed access to the outside, and are allowed to do what chickens and pigs are born to do, without the use of hormones or antibiotics. Some scientists have expressed concern that the widespread use of antibiotics in animals may be contributing to the emergence of antibiotic-resistant microbes. Many are likewise concerned with the effects that artificial hormones given to livestock may have on people.

There is no way of knowing which foods are GMOs or contain GMOs because there is no requirement in the United States for producers to label foods as such. GMOs that are already in our food supply include soybeans, corn, strawberries, canola oil, and potatoes. In addition, there are several new GMO foods that are currently up for review by the FDA to be released into our food system: wheat, alfalfa for livestock, and salmon. No one knows how the inserted genes will express themselves over time after they are ingested by people or animals. Some think the increased use of GMOs may be a contributing factor in the food allergies and intolerances that many people have.

---

## If You Had to Choose …

The Environmental Working Group, a nonprofit group monitoring pesticide use in the United States, lists the twelve conventionally grown fruits and vegetables that have the highest pesticide levels, on average. The group's "dirty dozen," updated every year, typically includes the following: apples, peaches, strawberries, nectarines, spinach, celery, grapes, bell peppers, cucumbers, potatoes, cherry tomatoes, and imported snap peas.

If you want to limit your exposure to synthetic chemicals such as pesticides, preservatives, and GMOs, especially for young children, opt for organic food whenever possible. Although I do not specifically call out each ingredient in my recipes as being organic, please assume that organic is the best option.

# BUDGETING FOR HEALTHY EATING

The first time you grocery shop after deciding to go grain-free, you'll probably notice an increase in cost at the checkout counter. If you were purchasing completely different foods than before cleaning up your diet, starting over with a grain-free and real-food pantry can be quite a task. Of course, the same is true for any "diet."

As being grain-free becomes a lifestyle, however, your grocery budget will eventually even out. You will notice that the bulk of your grocery list almost always comprises the same items: pasture-raised meats, eggs, and dairy; grain-free flours; organic vegetables and fruits; and herbs, spices, and occasionally a few condiments such as honey and coconut aminos. Below are a few suggestions for healthful eating on a budget.

**Turn the whole into parts.** One of my favorite methods for saving money is to use every last bit of what I buy. For example, I cook a whole chicken in the slow cooker nearly every week, use the schmaltz (fat/drippings) to cook with, and then turn the extra bits and bones into nourishing

bone both (page 93). Nothing goes to waste. And, by buying higher quality ingredients, you'll find that when you spend $15 on a whole chicken, you'll be even less likely to let any of it go to waste.

**Buy in bulk.** We all know that you can often get a cheaper price per pound when you buy in bulk. Whether it's meat or dry goods, it's the most effective way of maximizing your grocery budget. Keep in mind that you don't necessarily have to keep bulk purchases for yourself. Go in with a friend or even a group to split the cost.

**Buy direct.** When possible, cut out the middle-man. Buying meat, eggs, dairy, and produce directly from the farmer, instead of a grocery store, will give you a higher quality product and more bang for your buck. Consider starting with a CSA (community supported agriculture) program. There are CSAs for beef, chicken, pork, eggs, produce, and more. You'll pay for it up front, but you'll receive a weekly or biweekly portion for the duration of the season. Another option for produce is to pick your own from growers who follow organic practices. They often slash prices, since your labor time saves theirs. See page 199 for websites to get you started.

**Shop online.** Buying online is one of my favorite ways to shop, mostly because having things delivered to my front door saves tons of time. And it's so much easier to compare prices while sitting at home in your pajamas than it is running all over the neighborhood!

**Buy in season.** In-season produce is the most plentiful. So plentiful, in fact, that the price is reduced dramatically, and consumers will grab it up fast. If you have freezer space or like to can foods, stock up when fruits and veggies are at their rock-bottom prices, so you can eat from your surplus year-round.

**Choose frozen over fresh.** Farmers and manufactures freeze produce during peak season to make it available year-round. That's why you can often buy frozen fruits and vegetables for less than what you can get in the produce aisle.

**Grow your own.** I've been gardening since my early twenties, and it's something I enjoy doing, not only because it saves us money on our food budget but also because it's so rewarding to be able to feed my family from my own backyard. And once you start growing your own, you can save your seeds from year to year, another budgetary bonus. The tomato seeds my father-in-law saved from his tomatoes twenty years ago will continue filling my canning pantry for years.

**Keep meals simple.** You'll notice that the majority of the recipes in this book aren't very complicated. They all use similar, easy-to-find ingredients. Although I love to cook and enjoy being creative with the food I make, most often I keep our meals simple. But simple doesn't have to mean one-note or boring: typical weeknight dinners might include tossed salad, baked chicken thighs, buttered broccoli, and parsley potatoes; or kale salad, slow cooker beef roast, butternut squash puree, and green beans.

**Plan ahead.** Meal planning is key when keeping to your budget and sticking to your goals. At the end of each week, make a meal plan for the following week, and then write your shopping list around that meal plan. And stick to it.

# Chapter 3:

# GRAIN-FREE BASICS

LIKE A LOT OF PEOPLE, you might have found yourself relying on store-bought versions of basic foods. With premade pie crusts, biscuits in a can, pizza in a box, rice in a bag, and gravy in a jar readily available at every grocery store, you might have grown accustomed to their convenience. But when you decided to go grain-free, you may have been initially frustrated when there weren't grain-free options for these "convenience" foods. You might have even thought you'd have to give up these foods forever. And even if there was a grain-free recipe for what you wanted, the options can be so overwhelming that it's difficult to know where to start.

One of the most frustrating aspects of my transition to eating grain-free was when I'd pick up a grain-free cookbook and the bulk of the recipes were for things such as grilled chicken, tossed salads, or yogurt parfaits—foods that are naturally grain-free. There were no pastas, breadsticks, cereal, or muffins. As an extension of that experience, I decided that every single recipe I share will fill a void left by a grain-containing food.

What you won't find in this cookbook are recipes for foods that never had grain in them to begin with. You read that right: Each recipe in this book is my version of dishes that originally contained grains, whether obvious (such as manicotti) or hidden (such as creamed spinach). And unlike other grain-free cookbooks, my recipes aren't complicated or fancier renditions of traditional foods. I promise that they're easy to make even for those who are new to cooking. You're not going to find this combination anywhere else.

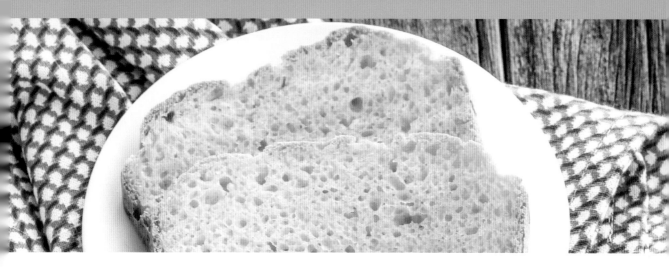

To get you started, I've created twelve amazing recipes that you'll find yourself making over and over. Most of them can be made ahead and frozen for quick reheating. In this chapter, you'll find recipes for foods that you thought you'd have to give up—such as Breadsticks (page 45) or Dinner Rolls (page 44)—or parts of a meal you thought you'd have to do without—such as Tortillas (page 41) or Breading Mix (page 34). Of course, I can't share every possible recipe you're looking for, but I've included many of the basics that I frequently turn to, all of which are adaptable to make new favorites. These recipes will also be used throughout the remaining chapters of this cookbook as key components or side dishes for other recipes, such as Buttermilk Biscuits in Creamed Chicken and Biscuits (page 123), Flat Bread in Greek Gyros with Tzatziki Sauce (page 144), and Cauliflower Rice in Cabbage Rolls in Tomato Sauce (page 118).

If you've never worked with grain-free ingredients before, you might be intimidated by them. Some of the recipes might seem like they would be difficult or challenging to perfect. Let me assure you that when you are cooking and baking with grain-free ingredients, you don't have to worry about clumping your sauces or overworking your biscuit or pasta doughs. In fact, with grain-free recipes, most often working your dough a little extra can help create an even better texture. There's also a lot less fuss.

So when you have a craving for a food from your grain-filled past, this is your place to start looking. Craving cinnamon-raisin bread? No worries, just add in some cinnamon and raisins to my Sliceable Sandwich Bread (page 38)! Experiment with the basic recipes in this chapter to help you adapt some of your own family favorites; that's how I turned pasta dough (page 37) into pierogi dough (page 138). You never know what kind of delicious creations you'll come up with!

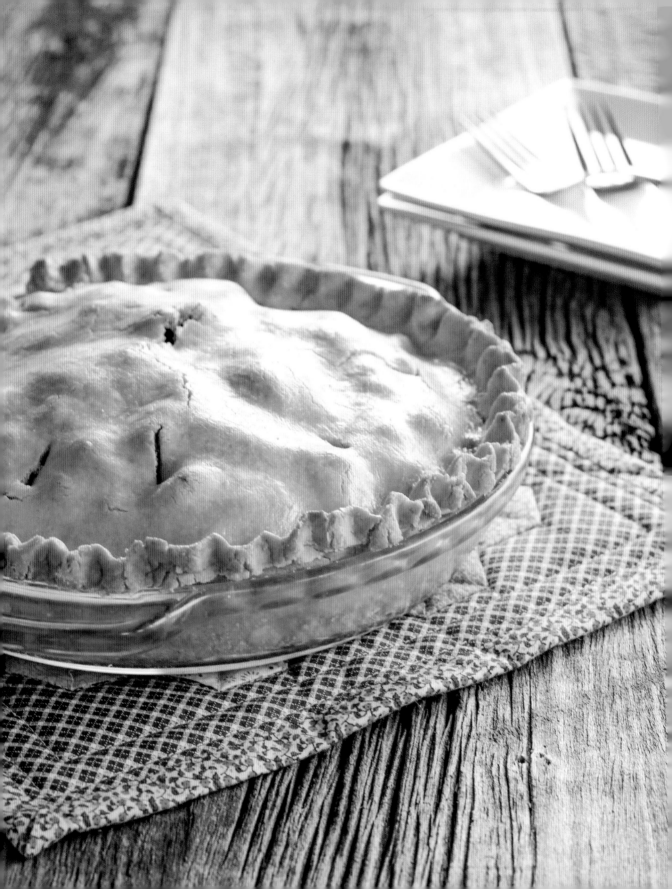

# PIE CRUST

This pie crust, although grain-free, is still buttery and flaky. It's perfect for any pie or tart, whether sweet pies such as Lemon Meringue Pie (page 174) or savory dinner pies such as Turkey Pot Pie (page 114).

1½ cups (168 g) blanched almond flour

1½ cups (180 g) tapioca starch

½ teaspoon baking powder (page 20)

½ teaspoon sea salt

1 large egg

¼ cup (55 g) butter, softened

1 teaspoon apple cider vinegar

Cold water, as needed

YIELD: ONE 9-INCH (23 CM) DOUBLE PIE CRUST OR 2 SINGLE CRUSTS

① Add the almond flour, tapioca starch, baking powder, and salt to the bowl of your food processor and pulse to mix.

② Add the egg, butter, and vinegar and pulse several times to combine. Continue pulsing until the dough holds together when pressed with your fingers. Add cold water, 1 teaspoon at a time as needed, if the dough will not come together.

③ Remove the dough from the food processor bowl and lightly knead until smooth. Use additional tapioca starch to prevent sticking.

④ Divide the dough into 2 equal portions and tightly wrap the unused portion in plastic wrap when not being used.

⑤ The dough can be carefully rolled out between 2 sheets of parchment paper or pressed into a pie plate using your fingers.

⑥ *For a prebaked, single pie crust:* Preheat the oven to 350°F (180°C, or gas mark 4) and bake for 15 minutes or until crispy.

NOTE  The dough can be stored in the fridge for up to 3 days or frozen for longer storage tightly wrapped with plastic wrap. (Freeze in half portions so you can take out what you need.) Allow frozen dough to thaw in the refrigerator overnight before using.

2 cups (224 g) blanched almond flour

2 cups (256 g) arrowroot starch

2 teaspoons sea salt

1 teaspoon garlic powder

1 teaspoon onion powder

1 teaspoon white pepper

YIELD: 4 CUPS (460 G)

# BREADING MIX

The possibilities for this simple breading mix are endless. I make up a double batch, keep it in a jar in the pantry, and take out just what I need. To make sure your breading sticks well to the food (when using any dry breading, not just this recipe), arrange the breaded food in a single layer on a wax paper–lined plate and freeze for at least an hour—I don't know how or why, but it works beautifully!

① In a large bowl, combine the flour, starch, salt, powders, and pepper and mix well.

② Store in an airtight container or plastic zip-top bag and use as needed in place of flour-based breading mixtures.

NOTE  This recipe can be halved or doubled as needed.

# CAULIFLOWER RICE

**1 large head of cauliflower**

## Yield: 6 to 8 cups (600 to 800 g)

It might seem odd at first, but when cauliflower is chopped into tiny pieces, it's the perfect substitution for rice as either an ingredient (Cabbage Rolls in Tomato Sauce, page 119) or a side dish (Indian Butter Chicken, page 148). The possibilities are endless.

① Remove any discolored spots from the head of cauliflower using a paring knife. Cut the head into quarters and remove the leaves and core. Coarsely chop or break the quarters into approximately 1-inch (2.5 cm) pieces.

② Working in batches, place the cauliflower pieces into a food processor and pulse several times to chop into rice-size pieces.

③ *Oven Cooking Method:* Preheat the oven to 425°F (220°C, or gas mark 7). Line a baking sheet with parchment paper. Spread a thin layer of cauliflower rice on the baking sheet. (Use a second sheet, if necessary, and switch or rotate the sheets halfway through baking.) Bake for 15 minutes, stirring halfway through. Remove and serve in place of cooked rice.

④ *Stove-Top Cooking Method:* Heat a large skillet over medium-high heat. Add a little cooking fat and cauliflower rice, stirring frequently to help release as much moisture as possible. When the rice is tender, after about 4 to 5 minutes, remove from the heat and serve in place of cooked rice.

⑤ *Freezer Storage:* Pack raw cauliflower rice into 1-quart (1 L) freezer bags, remove the air, and seal. Cauliflower rice can be stored in the freezer for up to 3 months. When preparing from frozen, allow to thaw slightly before cooking and then cook the same as from fresh.

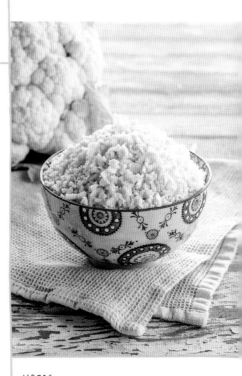

NOTES   Cooked Cauliflower Rice can be eaten plain as a side dish in place of rice with any meal, such as General Tso's Chicken (page 154). It can also be used to replace rice in recipes such as Ham and Shrimp Fried Rice (page 157) and Stuffed Peppers (page 112).

2 tablespoons (28 g) cooking fat or reserved pan drippings

3 tablespoons (36 g) potato starch or (32 g) arrowroot starch

¼ teaspoon garlic powder

¼ teaspoon onion powder

2 cups (475 ml) beef, chicken, or turkey broth or stock (preferably homemade, page 93)

2 tablespoons (28 ml) heavy cream

Sea salt and black pepper, to taste

YIELD: 2 CUPS (475 ML)

# GRAVY

We are chicken self-sufficient: Every spring on our homestead, in addition to our flock of twenty laying hens, we raise fifty free-range (meat) chickens, which yields enough chicken to last us a full year. One of our favorite meals is a simple roasted whole chicken, steamed broccoli, and mashed potatoes with this grain-free gravy, made thick and luscious with potato starch in place of all-purpose flour.

① In a medium saucepan, melt the fat over medium-high heat. Whisk in the potato starch, garlic powder, and onion powder.

② Whisking constantly, slowly add the broth. Continue to whisk until smooth and thickened, about 2 to 3 minutes.

③ Once the gravy is thickened, reduce the heat to low and gently stir in the cream. Continue to cook for 1 to 2 minutes or until heated through. Season with salt and pepper.

NOTES   The recipe can easily be halved or doubled as needed. If your gravy is not smooth, carefully transfer it to your blender and blend on high for 20 seconds or until completely smooth.

# PASTA DOUGH

Enjoy homemade noodles with the sauce of your choice or as a part of Fried Cabbage and Noodles (page 88), Home-Style Chicken Noodle Soup (page 107), Tuna Noodle Casserole (page 137), or Spaghetti and Meatballs (page 135). This pasta dough is also used in Potato and Cheese Pierogi (page 138) and Baked Manicotti (page 140).

1 cup (112 g) blanched almond flour

1 cup (120 g) tapioca starch

1 cup (128 g) arrowroot starch

2 teaspoons sea salt

3 large eggs

2 tablespoons (28 g) cooking fat, melted

2 tablespoons (28 ml) water

### YIELD: ABOUT 1 POUND (454 G) PASTA DOUGH (4 ADULT SERVINGS)

① In the bowl of a food processor or stand mixer fitted with a dough hook, add the flour, starches, and salt, and mix them until well combined.

② In a separate bowl, mix together the eggs, fat, and water. With the food processor or mixer running slowly, add the liquids into the dry ingredients. Continue running until the dough is a smooth ball. (Don't worry—you cannot overwork this dough because it's gluten-free.)

③ Remove the dough from the bowl and work in any remaining crumbs. This pasta can be rolled or extruded in a variety of pasta shapes. Use additional tapioca starch as needed to avoid sticking.

④ *Basic Homemade Noodles:* Divide the dough into 4 equal portions, lightly wrapping unused dough with plastic wrap. Dust your work surface and rolling pin with tapioca starch and roll out the dough as thinly as possible. Cut into the noodles using a knife or pizza cutter. Repeat for each portion of dough. (Use a dough scraper to pick up and move the noodles.)

⑤ Cook the noodles in plenty of boiling, salted water. The noodles will be done in 3 to 5 minutes, depending on their thickness. I recommend taste testing your noodles for doneness, as opposed to following a set time. Drain the cooked noodles and rinse with cold water to prevent sticking.

NOTES  The pasta dough can be made up to 1 day in advance and kept in the refrigerator wrapped tightly in plastic wrap. Allow the cold dough to warm slightly before working. Avoid making this recipe with an egg substitute.

- 1½ cups (144 g) blanched almond flour
- 1½ cups (183 g) tapioca starch
- 1½ cups (192 g) arrowroot starch
- 1 packet (2¼ teaspoons, or 7 g) active dry yeast
- 1 teaspoon sea salt
- 2 tablespoons (28 g) cooking fat, melted
- 2 teaspoons honey
- 1 large egg
- ¾ cup (180 ml) water, warmed to 100°F (38°C)

Yield: 1 loaf

# SLICEABLE SANDWICH BREAD

Here's a bread that can be used for sandwiches, toast, or as a side at dinner. Store the bread wrapped in a large plastic bag for 2 to 3 days at room temperature or 4 to 5 days in the refrigerator.

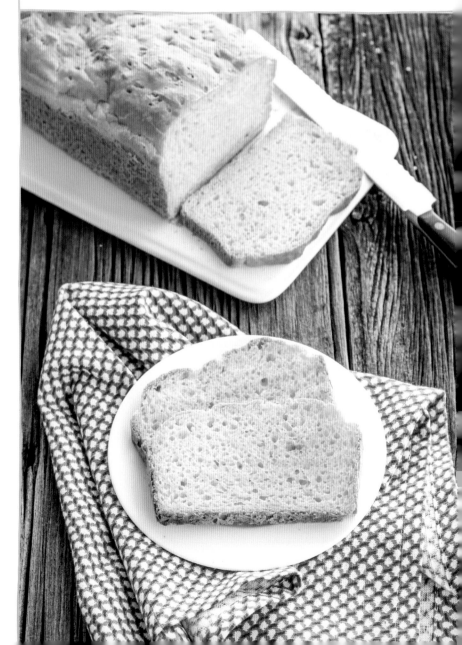

① In the bowl of a stand mixer fitted with the dough hook, combine the flour, starches, yeast, and salt on low speed.

② In a separate bowl, mix together the fat, honey, egg, and water. Slowly add this mixture to the dry ingredients while the machine is running. Once everything is mixed well, increase the speed to high and mix for 3 minutes. (The dough will be looser than gluten bread dough; this is normal.)

③ While the dough is mixing, turn the oven to 350°F (180°C, or gas mark 4) for exactly 2 minutes and then turn it off. (This creates a warm oven for the dough to rise in.)

④ Loosely cover the bowl of dough with plastic wrap and place in the warmed oven. Allow it to rise for 45 minutes, undisturbed.

⑤ Transfer the dough to a lightly greased 8½ x 4½-inch (21.6 x 11.4 cm) loaf pan, smoothing out the top with wet fingers. Preheat the oven (again) by heating to 350°F (180°C, or gas mark 4) for 2 minutes and then turn off the heat. Place the pan in the oven to rise for 30 minutes, undisturbed.

⑥ After 30 minutes, remove the dough and preheat the oven to 350°F (180°C, or gas mark 4).

⑦ Bake for 45 minutes until lightly brown and firm when tapped on top with your finger. Allow the bread to cool in the pan on a cooling rack for 15 minutes and then remove from the pan and allow to completely cool before slicing.

⑧ *For Croutons:* Cut leftover bread that is at least 1 day old into crouton-size cubes and then toss with a drizzle of melted butter and seasonings of your choice. Spread in a single layer on a parchment-lined cookie sheet and bake at 300°F (150°C, or gas mark 2), stirring often, for 10 to 15 minutes or until crispy. Croutons can be stored in an airtight container for up to 1 week.

⑨ *For Bread Crumbs:* Cut leftover bread that is at least 1 day old into 1-inch (2.5 cm) cubes, place in the food processor, and pulse to make into crumbs (seasonings and dried herbs can be added as desired). Use as fresh bread crumbs immediately or dry in a low 200°F (93°C) oven for an hour, or until crispy. Store the bread crumbs in the refrigerator for up to a week or in the freezer for up to 3 months. Use in place of traditional bread crumbs in any recipe.

NOTES  Sliced bread can be stored in the freezer for up to 3 months in a sealed bag or container. Allow it to thaw at room temperature before using. Frozen bread slices are best used for toast and heated sandwiches (such as grilled cheese).

The dough can be shaped into buns or rolls after the initial rise using liberal amounts of additional tapioca starch to make it less tacky and easier to handle.

½ cup (56 g) blanched almond flour

½ cup (60 g) tapioca starch

½ teaspoon garlic powder

½ teaspoon onion powder

½ teaspoon sea salt

¼ teaspoon white pepper

½ cup (120 ml) water

Cooking fat

YIELD: 4 FLAT BREADS

# FLAT BREAD

These grain-free flat breads have been one of my most popular recipes on *Health Starts in the Kitchen*. They are so easy and versatile. When we are short on time and need a quick meal, we use these flatbreads to make individual pizzas.

① Preheat the oven to 350°F (180°C, or gas mark 4) and line a baking sheet with parchment paper.

② In a medium bowl, combine the flour, starch, powders, salt, pepper, and water. Mix well to make a thin batter.

③ Heat a nonstick skillet over medium heat and add a little bit of fat to the pan.

④ Pour approximately ¼ cup (55 g) of batter into the skillet and cook for 1 to 2 minutes per side or just until each side develops a few brown spots. Flat breads will be firm on the outside but uncooked in the center.

⑤ Transfer the flat breads to the baking sheet. Continue making flat breads until the batter is used up.

⑥ Bake for 10 to 15 minutes. Less time will result in a softer bread; more time will result in a crispier bread. Remove from the oven and cool slightly before serving.

⑦ These breads are especially good served with Spinach and Artichoke Dip (page 70), as a wrap for Greek Gyros with Tzatziki Sauce (page 144), or with Indian Butter Chicken (page 148).

NOTES  The recipe can be made in larger batches as needed. After cooking the flat breads in a skillet, freeze them for up to 3 months. Allow the frozen flat breads to thaw slightly and then bake as directed.

# TORTILLAS

Tex-Mex and Mexican foods are delicious and simple to make—they're perfect for quick weeknight dinners. And with this recipe, you don't need to give them up, even when eating grain-free! These soft and delicious tortillas are great for making into Tortilla Chips (page 82), Southwest Quesadillas (page 78), or crispy taco shells (page 146).

½ cup (56 g) blanched almond flour

½ cup (64 g) arrowroot starch

½ teaspoon sea salt

¼ teaspoon turmeric (optional)

2 tablespoons (28 g) cooking fat, softened

1 to 2 tablespoons (15 to 28 ml) water

Yield: 4 tortillas

① Combine the flour, starch, and salt using a food processor or mixer. Add the turmeric, if desired, for yellow, corn-style tortillas or Crispy Beef Tacos (page 146).

② Add the fat and pulse until a coarse meal forms. Add 1 tablespoon (15 ml) of water and pulse several times. If the dough does not come together around the blade, add the remaining 1 tablespoon (15 ml) water.

③ Using additional arrowroot starch as needed, remove the dough from the bowl, work into a large-size ball, and then divide into 4 equal portions. Roll each portion into a ball and use a tortilla press lined with plastic wrap that has been dusted with arrowroot starch to press each ball into a tortilla. If you do not have a tortilla press, roll out the dough between layers of plastic wrap with a rolling pin.

④ Cook each tortilla in a preheated, ungreased cast-iron skillet over medium heat for 1 to 2 minutes per side or until each develops a few light brown spots. Stack cooked tortillas on a plate and loosely cover with a cotton towel. Repeat with the remaining dough. (These tortillas can be used in place of flour tortillas in any recipe.)

NOTE   Cooked tortillas will keep, covered, in the fridge for up to 3 days or in the freezer for up to 6 months. Allow them to thaw before using.

**2 tablespoons (28 g) cooking fat**

**2 tablespoons (21 g) arrowroot starch**

**1 teaspoon dry mustard powder**

**1 cup (235 ml) milk**

**2 cups (225 g) shredded Cheddar cheese**

**Sea salt, to taste**

YIELD: 2 CUPS (475 ML)

# CHEESE SAUCE

Traditional cheese sauces typically start with a roux—equal parts fat and flour—to thicken them. My version does away with the grain but retains all the creaminess and richness. For a special treat, top a baked potato with cubes of leftover chicken, steamed broccoli, and this creamy cheese sauce for a family-friendly meal.

① In a medium-size saucepan over medium heat, melt the fat. Whisk in the arrowroot starch and mustard powder until combined. Slowly add in the milk, whisking constantly.

② Remove from the heat and add the cheese, whisking constantly until smooth. Add salt to taste.

NOTE   Add diced jalapeño pepper for a spicy nacho cheese sauce and serve with Tortilla Chips (page 82).

# BUTTERMILK BISCUITS

These biscuits are best eaten within a few hours of baking. My husband's favorite impromptu dessert is one of these biscuits, served warm, with a generous pat of butter and a drizzle of local honey.

① Preheat the oven to 350°F (180°C, or gas mark 4) and line a baking sheet with parchment paper.

② Combine the flour, starch, baking soda, salt, and baking powder in a large bowl. Add 3 tablespoons (42 g) of the butter, buttermilk, and eggs to the dry ingredients and mix until completely combined into a smooth dough.

③ Using your hands dusted with additional arrowroot starch, divide the dough into 8 equal portions and form into biscuit shapes.

④ Place each biscuit 1 to 2 inches (2.5 to 5 cm) apart on the baking sheet and bake for 10 minutes. Baste each biscuit with the remaining 2 tablespoons (28 g) melted butter and then bake for an additional 10 minutes.

⑤ Transfer the biscuits to a rack and allow to cool.

**2½ cups (280 g) blanched almond flour**

**⅓ cup (43 g) arrowroot starch**

**½ teaspoon baking soda**

**½ teaspoon sea salt**

**¼ teaspoon baking powder (page 20)**

**5 tablespoons (70 g) butter, melted, divided**

**¼ cup (60 ml) cultured buttermilk (or ¼ cup [60 ml] whole milk and ¾ teaspoon apple cider vinegar)**

**2 large eggs, beaten**

## Yield: 8 biscuits

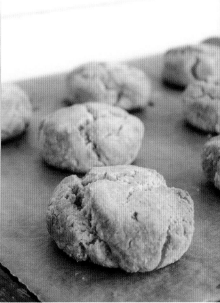

NOTE   Baked biscuits can be frozen and reheated in a 300°F (150°C, or gas mark 2) oven for about 10 minutes.

1 cup (120 g) tapioca starch

¼ cup (32 g) arrowroot starch

⅓ cup (37 g) coconut flour

1 teaspoon sea salt

1 large egg

½ cup (112 g) cooking fat, melted

½ cup (120 ml) water

1 teaspoon honey

Yield: 8 rolls

# DINNER ROLLS

Crusty on the outside, while soft and delicate on the inside, these simple dinner rolls will fool even the pickiest of eaters. Most often, I make them with "everything," rolling them in a mixture of garlic powder, poppy seeds, and sesame seeds prior to baking.

① Preheat the oven to 325°F (170°C, or gas mark 3) and line a baking sheet with parchment paper.

② In a medium-size bowl, whisk together the starches, flour, and salt. In a separate bowl, mix together the egg, fat, water, and honey. Add the liquids to the dry ingredients and stir until well combined into a smooth dough.

③ Divide the dough into 8 equal portions and roll each section into a ball, using additional arrowroot starch to keep the dough from sticking to your fingers.

④ Place each ball on the prepared baking sheet and bake for 40 minutes. For best results, allow the rolls to cool before serving.

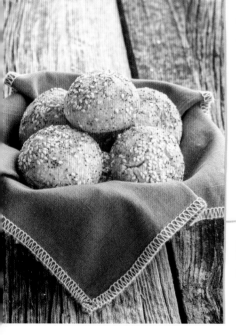

NOTE  Baked rolls can be frozen and reheated in a 300°F (150°C, or gas mark 2) oven for about 10 minutes.

# BREADSTICKS (GRISSINI)

These thin and crispy breadsticks are the prefect addition to a traditional Italian-style meal or can be eaten with dips in place of crackers. For a special treat, use this dough to completely cover mozzarella string cheese sticks and bake at 350°F (180°C, or gas mark 4) for 15 minutes for a soft, cheese-filled breadstick.

1½ cups (168 g) blanched almond flour

1 tablespoon (11 g) potato flour

1 cup (120 g) tapioca starch

1 teaspoon garlic powder

1 teaspoon onion powder

1 teaspoon sea salt

½ teaspoon white pepper

1 large egg

⅓ cup (80 ml) water

1 tablespoon (14 g) cooking fat

YIELD: 2 DOZEN 12-INCH (30 CM) BREADSTICKS

① Preheat the oven to 350°F (180°C, or gas mark 4) and line a baking sheet with parchment paper.

② Combine the flours, starch, powders, salt, pepper, egg, water, and fat in a food processor and process until it forms a smooth dough.

③ Divide the dough into 24 pieces. Roll each piece into a ½-inch (1.3 cm)-diameter log and place on the prepared baking sheet. Bake for 20 to 25 minutes, or until crisp, rolling over halfway through baking. If all of the breadsticks do not fit on one baking sheet, bake in multiple batches.

④ Allow to cool completely on a wire rack. Breadsticks can be stored in an airtight container for up to a week.

NOTE   The breadsticks can be sprinkled with sesame seeds, poppy seeds, and/or garlic powder prior to baking.

# Chapter 4:

# BREAKFASTS

BREAKFAST is an important meal, though unfortunately for many people, it usually consists of sugar and carbohydrates. The problem with a grain- and sugar-laden breakfast is that it will leave you feeling depleted and hungry just a couple hours after eating because your blood sugar levels will surge and then rapidly fall. Starting the day with healthy fats from butter, eggs, and bacon will satiate the body and give it the fuel it needs to work throughout the morning. Many people find that when they eat a nourishing breakfast devoid of grain and full of healthy fats and adequate protein, they aren't even hungry when lunchtime comes.

If you were around for the low-fat diet craze of the '90s, you may have found yourself convinced that fat is the enemy. But that's not necessarily true.

Fat is actually a vital nutrient. It helps carry essential nutrients throughout your body and serves as a reserve for energy storage. Fat supplies essential fatty acids necessary for growth, healthy skin, vitamin absorption, and regulation of bodily functions. Eating enough fat may actually help you manage your weight by providing a better sense of satiety than other, lower-fat foods. In fact, eating too little fat is associated with a number of health problems, such as depression and an increased risk of cancer. So, try not to think of fat as your mortal diet enemy, but rather as a helpful counterpart in the pursuit of your healthier lifestyle!

Foods with a higher fat content truly are more satisfying than their low-fat counterparts. When you're hungry and you eat only low-fat foods, that gnawing hunger never really goes away. When you eat just enough fat, the sense of satisfaction will obliterate that ever-present hunger pang. The reason is that fat actually takes longer to digest than some other types of foods. Because it sticks around in your stomach a while, you'll feel fuller longer and be less inclined to eat until you feel a sense of hunger again. For example, if you eat an egg white omelet with low-fat cheese in the morning, your tummy may grumble by the time you've settled into your cubicle; by simply leaving in the nutrient-rich yolks and using full-fat cheese, that morning meal will have longer staying power.

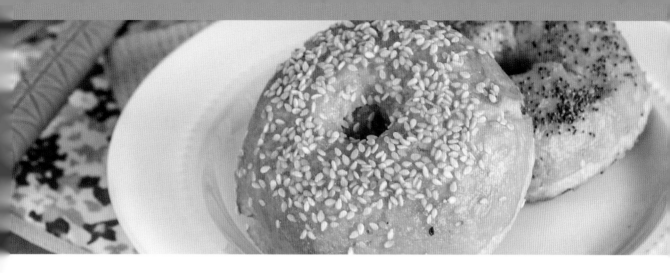

It's always best to pair your occasional indulgent (carbohydrate-heavy) breakfasts with adequate protein and healthy fats. Adding a side of sausage and a pat of butter with your waffles, topping your bagel with cream cheese and smoked salmon, or treating a decadent cinnamon roll as a breakfast dessert after eggs and bacon will help minimize the effects of the sugar and carbohydrates on blood sugar levels.

Although juicing and smoothies are growing in popularity as a quick breakfast, it's important to remember that fruits and vegetables contain fat-soluble vitamins, which can only be absorbed when consumed with fats. Aside from being delicious, blending half an avocado and a couple of raw egg yolks into your morning juice or smoothie will help make it into a more balanced meal. Another way to ensure you're getting all your essential fats and protein for breakfast is having a Bulletproof coffee (also known as butter coffee). Using your blender to blend unsalted butter, coconut oil, and collagen peptides (a source of easily digestible protein made from

grass-fed animals) into hot black coffee will produce a surprisingly creamy, frothy coffee that's full of healthy fats and protein. On hurried mornings, it's my go-to breakfast that will keep me satisfied and full of energy until lunch and most often beyond.

Usually, my family has quick and simple breakfasts during the week. Eggs are our favorite way to start the day. In addition to being a healthy source of fat, they're loaded with protein and vitamin D, plus hard-to-get choline, a nutrient that may curb anxiety and boost memory. On weekends, I make up a bunch of hard-boiled eggs, sausage links, and bacon and package them in convenient baggies that are perfect for grab-and-go breakfasts, along with a warm mug of bone broth (page 93) or a green juice, before work or school. However, on the weekends, we enjoy bigger, indulgent breakfasts, including Crispy Belgian Waffles (page 49), Bagels (page 50), and, on special occasions, Cinnamon Rolls (page 60). With choices such as these, you'll never want to skip breakfast!

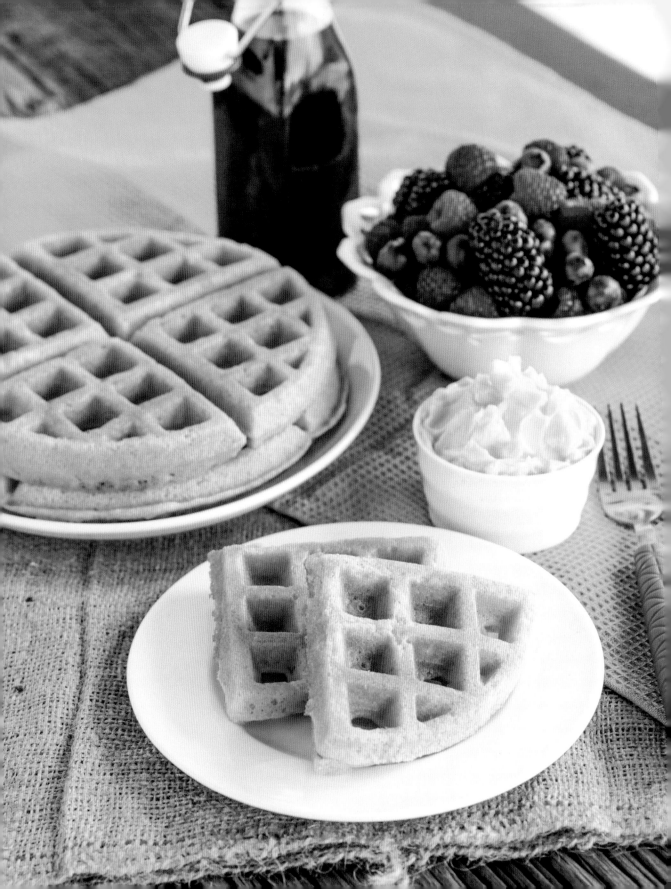

# CRISPY BELGIAN WAFFLES

If you want to convince your friends and family that grain-free cooking can be every bit as delicious as cooking with grains, then this is your recipe! If you're like me and love your waffles with lots of butter, instead of spreading butter directly on the waffles, combine equal parts of butter and maple syrup in a small-size saucepan over low heat until the butter is melted. Drizzle the butter maple syrup over your freshly made Belgian waffles just before eating.

2 cups (224 g) blanched almond flour

1 cup (120 g) tapioca starch

¼ cup (60 g) coconut sugar

4 teaspoons (10 g) baking powder (page 20)

½ teaspoon sea salt

2 large eggs

1 cup (235 ml) milk

½ cup (112 g) cooking fat, melted

Juice of ½ of a lemon

1 teaspoon vanilla extract

YIELD: 4 LARGE-SIZE WAFFLES

(1) Preheat a waffle iron according to the manufacturer's directions.

(2) In a large bowl, whisk together the flour, starch, sugar, baking powder, and salt. In a smaller bowl, mix together the eggs, milk, fat, lemon juice, and vanilla. Add the wet ingredients to the dry and mix gently until combined. It is okay if there are a few lumps.

(3) Scoop or pour one-quarter of the batter into the hot waffle iron and close the lid. Cook the waffles according to the manufacturer's instructions. For extra-crispy waffles, extend the cooking time in the waffle maker until the desired level of crispiness is achieved. Serve immediately or cool on a wire rack (so they stay crisp).

NOTE   Cooled waffles can be frozen and reheated in the toaster for quick breakfasts.

**3 cups (336 g) blanched almond flour**

**1 cup (120 g) tapioca starch**

**2 teaspoons sea salt**

**2 teaspoons baking powder (page 20)**

**⅔ cup (160 ml) warm water**

**2 tablespoons (28 ml) apple cider vinegar**

**2 tablespoons (40 g) honey**

**1 egg yolk, beaten**

**Optional toppings: toasted onion flakes, garlic powder, poppy seeds, sesame seeds, etc.**

YIELD: 6 TO 8 BAGELS

# BAGELS

These bagels are boiled and then baked for that authentic bagel flavor and texture. They can be topped with coarse salt, sesame seeds, poppy seeds, toasted onion flakes, or all of these just before baking. And don't forget to smear with cultured cream cheese or butter and jelly!

① Preheat the oven to 350°F (180°C, or gas mark 4). Line a baking sheet with parchment paper.

② In a large pot over high heat, bring about 4 inches (10 cm) of water to a boil. Add a pinch of sea salt.

③ In a large bowl, combine the flour, starch, salt, and baking powder. Add the water, vinegar, and honey and mix well.

④ Divide the dough into 6 to 8 equal portions. Dust your hands with additional tapioca starch and roll each section of dough into a ball. Flatten the ball and use your finger to push through the center to make a bagel shape. Place each bagel onto the baking sheet.

⑤ Working in batches of 3 or 4 bagels, carefully place each bagel into the boiling water for 1 minute (or until they float). Using a slotted spoon, remove them from the water and place them back onto the baking sheet.

⑥ Bake the boiled bagels for 10 minutes. Remove from the oven, brush with the beaten egg yolk, and top as desired. Return to the oven and bake for an additional 10 minutes.

⑦ After baking for a total of 20 minutes, increase the temperature of the oven to 425°F (220°C, or gas mark 7) and bake for 5 additional minutes or until lightly browned and crispy.

⑧ Transfer the bagels to a rack and allow to cool.

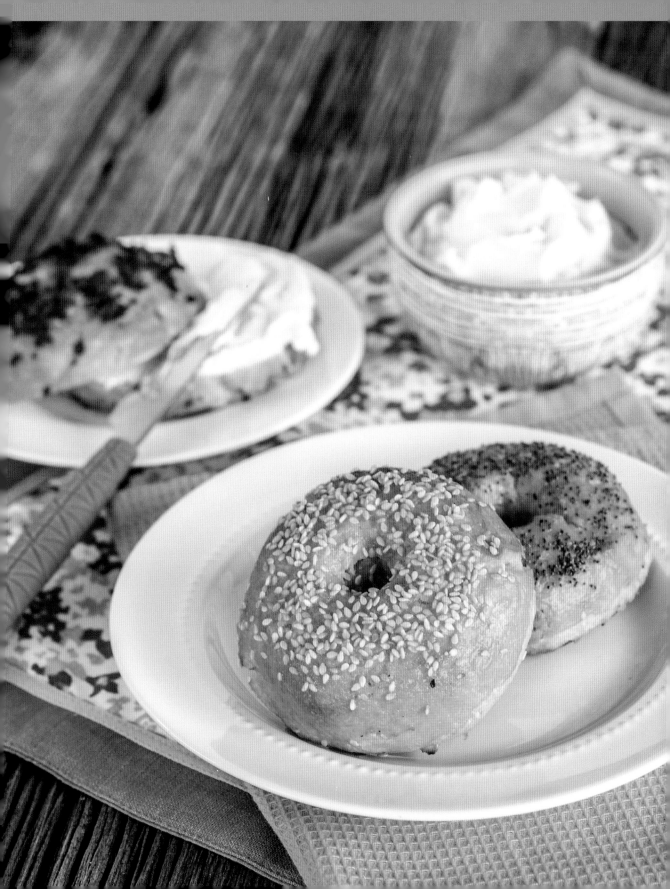

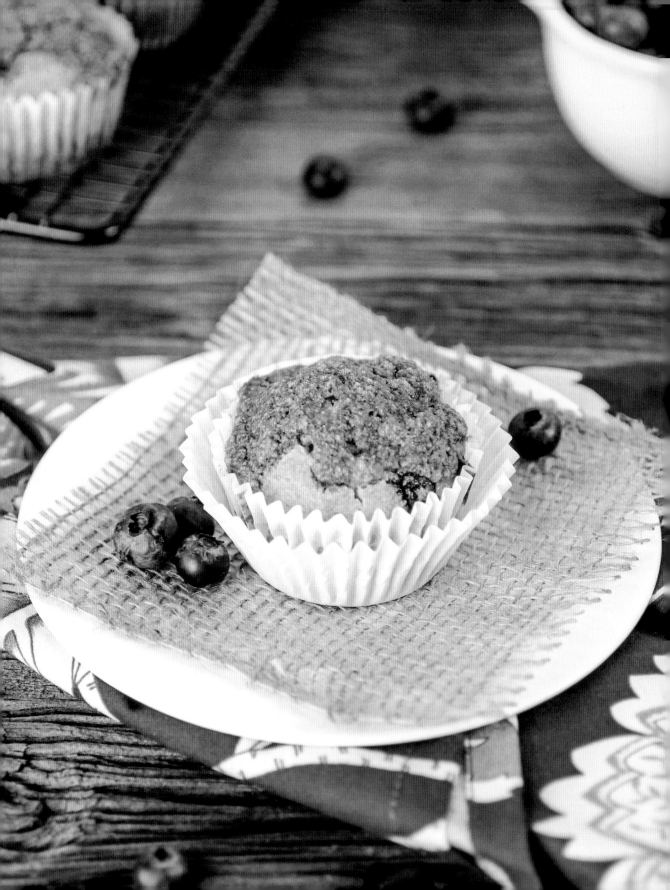

# BLUEBERRY MUFFINS WITH CRUMB TOPPING

Not just for breakfast, these blueberry-loaded muffins with a cinnamon-sugar crumb topping are best served warm with a generous pat of butter. If you aren't in the mood for blueberry, swap them for cranberries and add fresh orange zest for a special sweet and sour treat.

① Preheat the oven to 350°F (180°C, or gas mark 4) and line a 12-cup muffin pan with paper liners.

② To make the muffins: In a large bowl, combine the flour, starch, cinnamon, baking powder, and salt. In a separate small bowl or mixing cup, combine the eggs, honey, and vanilla. Add the wet mixture to the dry ingredients, mixing just enough to combine, and then gently fold in the blueberries.

③ To make the topping: In a small bowl, use your fingers to crumble together the topping ingredients.

④ Divide the muffin batter evenly among 12 muffin cups. Top each with crumb topping. Bake for 35 to 40 minutes or until a toothpick inserted into the center comes out clean. As soon as the muffins are cool enough to handle, transfer them to a rack and allow to cool before serving.

## FOR MUFFINS:

2½ cups (280 g) blanched almond flour

½ cup (64 g) arrowroot starch

½ teaspoon ground cinnamon

½ teaspoon baking powder (page 20)

½ teaspoon sea salt

3 large eggs

⅓ cup (107 g) honey

1 teaspoon vanilla extract

1 cup (145 g) fresh or (155 g) frozen blueberries

## FOR CRUMB TOPPING:

¼ cup (28 g) blanched almond flour

¼ cup (32 g) arrowroot starch

¼ cup (55 g) cooking fat, softened

¼ cup (48 g) coconut sugar

½ teaspoon ground cinnamon

Pinch of sea salt

### YIELD: 12 MUFFINS

1 pound (455 g) bulk sausage (breakfast, country, or sage-seasoned)

¼ cup (48 g) potato starch

½ teaspoon onion powder

¼ teaspoon garlic powder

⅛ teaspoon paprika

⅛ teaspoon ground sage

3 cups (700 ml) milk

Sea salt and black pepper, to taste

4 Buttermilk Biscuits (page 43), halved

YIELD: 4 SERVINGS

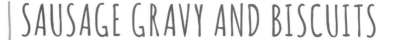

# SAUSAGE GRAVY AND BISCUITS

No one will leave the table hungry after a breakfast of grain-free biscuits and this hearty Southern-style sausage gravy. Serve topped with a sunny-side-up egg and side of fried potatoes.

① In a 2-quart (2 L) saucepan over medium-high heat, cook the sausage, using a spatula to break up any large pieces. Add the starch, powders, paprika, and sage and cook for 1 minute.

② Reduce the heat to low. Add the milk, whisking until the gravy is without clumps of starch. Continue to simmer until thickened. Season to taste with salt and pepper.

③ Serve each person 2 biscuit halves topped with one-fourth of the gravy.

NOTES   These sausages can also be served over toasted bread (page 38) instead of biscuits. Using this same method, you can make creamed chip beef by using chopped dried beef in place of the sausage.

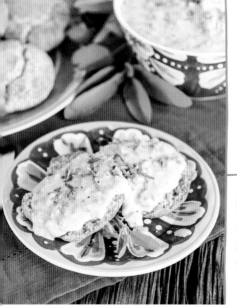

# FLUFFY PANCAKES

There's no way I could leave pancakes out of this book!
They make up one of our favorite lazy Sunday morning
breakfasts, served with lots of butter, a generous drizzle
of maple syrup, and country sausage patties.

① Preheat the oven to 200°F (93°C) or other "warm" setting.

② In a large bowl, whisk together the eggs, water, and vanilla.
Add the flour, starches, sugar, baking powder, baking soda, and
salt. Whisk until the batter is well combined.

③ Heat a griddle or seasoned cast-iron skillet over medium
heat, and then add the fat. Working in batches, pour ¼ cup (55 g)
batter for each pancake onto the griddle. Cook until the surface
is bubbling and the edges are slightly dry, about 2 to 3 minutes.
Turn the pancakes over; cook until the undersides are golden
brown, about 2 to 3 minutes more. Transfer to a baking sheet,
and keep warm in the oven. Serve with maple syrup and butter,
if desired.

6 large eggs, beaten

1½ cups (355 ml) water

2 teaspoons vanilla extract

1 cup (112 g) coconut flour

½ cup (60 g) tapioca starch

½ cup (64 g) arrowroot starch

2 tablespoons (24 g) coconut
sugar

1 teaspoon baking powder
(page 20)

1 teaspoon baking soda

¼ teaspoon sea salt

1 tablespoon (14 g) cooking
fat

**Maple syrup and butter, for
topping**

## Yield: Ten 4-inch (10 cm) pancakes

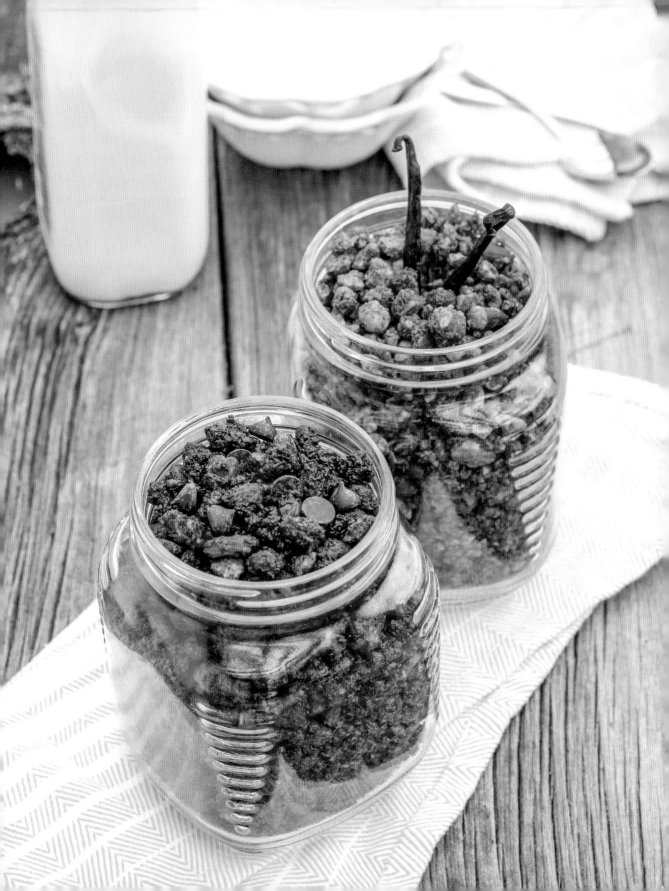

# VANILLA OR DARK CHOCOLATE GRANOLA

Make extra batches of this honey-sweetened, nutty granola so you'll have some on hand for quick breakfasts and snacks. We especially enjoy this granola along with cultured yogurt and fresh-picked raspberries in July.

1 Preheat the oven to 350°F (180°C, or gas mark 4) and line a baking sheet with parchment paper.

2 In a food processor, working in batches, coarsely chop the nuts into pea-size pieces. Transfer to a large bowl. Add the coconut, salt, and cinnamon and stir to combine. In a separate smaller bowl, combine the honey, oil, and vanilla. Add the wet ingredients to the dry and mix well. Toss with the sugar.

3 Spread the granola mixture in a thin layer on the baking sheet and bake for about 30 minutes, stirring every 5 minutes. You want your granola to *toast*, so remove it from the oven as soon as it starts to brown.

4 For dark chocolate granola, quickly sprinkle the chocolate chips over the hot granola and mix well. The residual heat from the granola and pan will melt them. Continue to mix until all the chips are melted and combined with the granola.

5 Store the granola in an airtight container for several weeks. Serve with milk or yogurt.

3 cups raw nuts, such as (435 g) almonds, (420 g) cashews, (300 g) pecans, or (300 g) walnuts (preferably soaked, see Note)

1 cup (85 g) shredded unsweetened coconut

1½ teaspoons sea salt

1 teaspoon ground cinnamon

½ cup (160 g) honey

3 tablespoons (42 g) coconut oil, melted

1 teaspoon vanilla extract

¼ cup (48 g) coconut sugar

Optional: 1 cup (175 g) dark chocolate chips

YIELD: 8 CUPS (1.2 KG)

NOTE  Raw nuts are healthiest when soaked overnight in filtered water and then drained and dehydrated prior to eating. This recipe will work fine without soaking first.

2 tablespoons (24 g) cane
    sugar

4 teaspoons (9 g) ground
    cinnamon, divided

½ cup (56 g) blanched
    almond flour

½ cup (60 g) tapioca starch

¼ cup (48 g) coconut sugar

1 teaspoon vanilla extract

3 tablespoons (42 g) coconut
    oil, melted

1 large egg

2 tablespoons (28 ml) water

YIELD: 4 CUPS (600 G)

# HOMEMADE CINNAMON CRUNCH CEREAL

After making this grain-free cereal, you won't crave
the boxed variety again! It's easy to make and full of
cinnamon flavor. Be sure to bake the flakes until very crisp
so that they will not get soggy too quickly in the milk.

① Preheat the oven to 325°F (170°C, or gas mark 3).

② In a small-size bowl or shaker, combine the cane sugar and
1 tablespoon (7 g) of the cinnamon. Set aside.

③ In a food processor, combine the flour, starch, coconut sugar,
remaining 1 teaspoon (2 g) cinnamon, vanilla, oil, egg, and water.
Process until a smooth dough is formed. Add additional water,
1 teaspoon at a time, if needed, to form a dough.

④ Roll out the dough between 2 pieces of parchment paper into an
8 x 12-inch (20 x 30.5-cm) rectangle. Transfer the parchment and
dough to a baking sheet and remove the top layer of parchment.

⑤ Using a pizza cutter or knife, score the dough into ¾-inch (2 cm)
squares (the pieces will not be separated yet). Sprinkle with the
reserved cinnamon-sugar topping.

⑥ Bake for 10 minutes, remove from the oven, and recut on the
same lines as before baking. Return to the oven and bake for an
additional 10 to 15 minutes or until the pieces are crispy.

⑦ Carefully transfer the cereal, on the parchment, onto a cooling
rack and allow to cool completely before eating. The cereal can be
stored in an airtight container for several weeks.

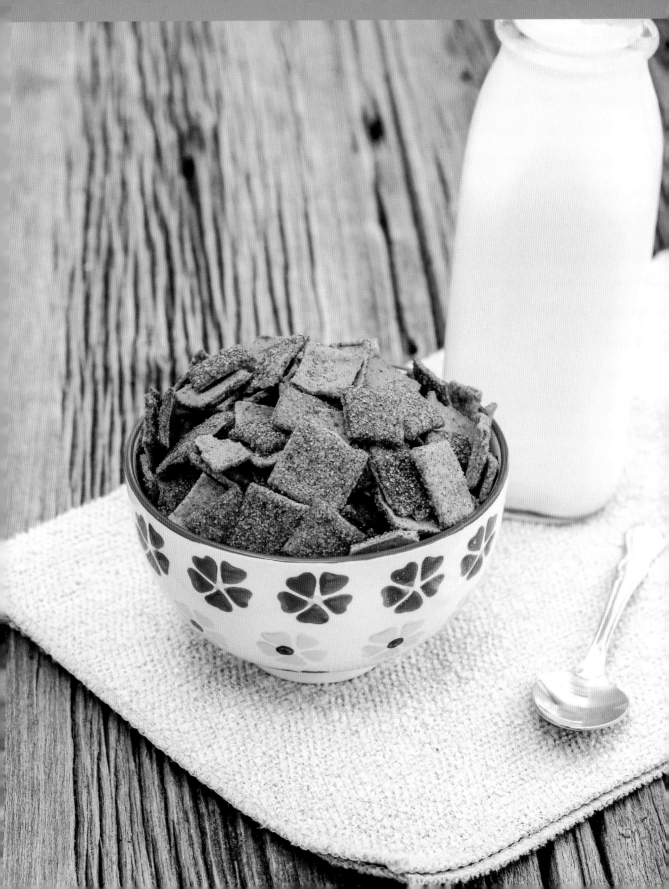

## FOR DOUGH:

1 packet (2¼ teaspoons, or 7 g) active dry yeast

¼ cup (48 g) cane sugar

⅔ cup (160 ml) milk

¼ cup (60 g) melted butter, divided

½ cup (56 g) blanched almond flour

½ cup (96 g) potato starch

½ cup (64 g) arrowroot starch

¼ cup (30 g) tapioca starch, plus more for flouring your surface

2½ teaspoons baking powder (page 20)

1 teaspoon powdered gelatin

½ teaspoon baking soda

½ teaspoon sea salt

1 large egg

½ teaspoon vanilla extract

## FOR FILLING:

⅓ cup (75 g) butter, softened

½ cup (96 g) coconut sugar

2 tablespoons (14 g) ground cinnamon

## FOR ICING:

¾ cup (90 g) powdered sugar

3 tablespoons (42 g) butter, softened

2 tablespoons (30 g) cream cheese, softened

½ teaspoon vanilla extract

Pinch of sea salt

YIELD: 8 CINNAMON ROLLS

# CINNAMON ROLLS

Everyone loves a cinnamon roll. Soft and fluffy, filled with a cinnamon swirl and topped with ooey-gooey cream cheese frosting, these rolls will make you fall in love at first bite! You can even make them months ahead of time. Once the rolls are arranged in the pie plate, cover securely with plastic wrap and freeze. Allow them to thaw overnight in the fridge and set them out to rise for at least 25 minutes before baking.

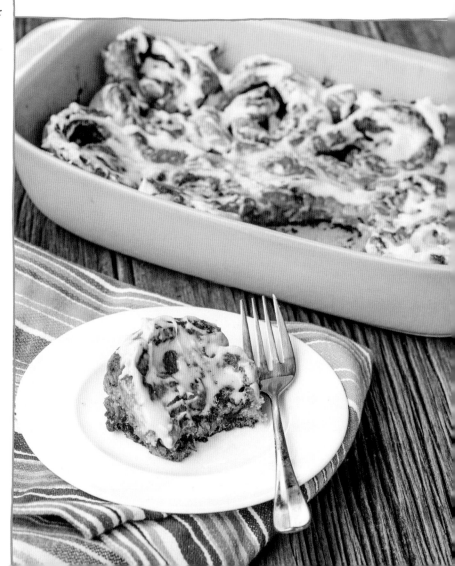

① To make the dough: Combine the yeast and sugar in a large mixing bowl or the bowl of a stand mixer.

② Heat the milk and 1 tablespoon (14 g) of the butter to 110° to 115°F (43° to 46°C). Whisk into the yeast mixture until the yeast granules are dissolved and set aside until foaming, about 5 to 10 minutes.

③ Meanwhile, in a small bowl, whisk together the flour, starches, baking powder, gelatin, baking soda, and salt.

④ Once the yeast is foamy, add in the egg, the remaining 3 tablespoons (42 g) butter, and the vanilla. Mix, using a hand or stand mixer, for a moment and then slowly add in the flour mixture. Turn the mixer up to medium-high and beat for 2 minutes. The dough will thicken and lose its stickiness as you beat it.

⑤ Cover a work surface with 2 large pieces of plastic wrap and dust with a light layer of tapioca starch. Place the dough in the center and cover with a bit more tapioca starch and another sheet (or two) of plastic wrap. Roll the dough out to approximately a 13 x 10-inch (33 x 25 cm) rectangle and then carefully peel off the top layer of plastic wrap. (It is a very sticky dough.)

⑥ To make the filling: Using a knife or spatula, gently spread the butter over the dough, leaving an even, ½-inch (1.3 cm) border around the edges.

⑦ In a small bowl, combine the sugar and cinnamon. Sprinkle evenly over the butter.

⑧ Starting at a short side, roll the dough into a log. Use the plastic wrap to help you "lift and roll" the dough as you go along. Try to make it a nice tight roll, but do not try to unroll it and redo it. You'll end up with a sticky mess.

⑨ Dip a sharp knife into tapioca starch and then cut the log into 8 pieces. Place the rolls, cut-side down, in a greased pie plate (it is okay if they touch each other).

⑩ Preheat the oven to 350°F (180°C, or gas mark 4) for exactly 2 minutes and then turn off the heat. This will create a warm oven for the dough to rise in.

⑪ Place the rolls in the warmed oven and let them rise for 30 minutes, undisturbed.

⑫ Remove the rolls from the oven and preheat it to 350°F (180°C, or gas mark 4). Bake for 25 minutes or until the top is golden brown.

⑬ To make the icing: While the rolls are in the oven, prepare the icing. In a mixing bowl, beat the sugar, butter, and cream cheese until smooth. Beat in the vanilla and salt.

⑭ Drizzle the icing over the tops of the cinnamon rolls as soon as they come out of the oven.

NOTE  For easy breakfast cinnamon rolls, once they're in the pie plate, cover with plastic wrap and place in the fridge. In the morning, set them out for at least 25 minutes before baking.

- 3 cups roasted, unsalted nuts ([435 g] almonds, [420 g] cashews, [300 g] pecans, [300 g] walnuts), or a combination, coarsely chopped
- 1 cup dried fruit ([130 g] apricots, [114 g] mango, [120 g] cranberries, [145 g] raisins, [120 g] pineapple), or a combination, coarsely chopped
- 1 tablespoon (12 g) flaxseeds
- ⅓ cup (107 g) honey
- ⅓ cup (80 ml) maple syrup
- ¼ teaspoon sea salt
- 1 teaspoon vanilla extract
- Optional: 1 cup (175 g) dark chocolate chips

Yield: 20 Granola bars

# GRANOLA BARS

Not only are store-bought granola bars full of grains and preservatives, but they also are expensive. By making your own, you have complete control over the ingredients and can buy your supplies in bulk to save money. Feel free to experiment with different flavor combinations and create a granola bar that's perfect for you.

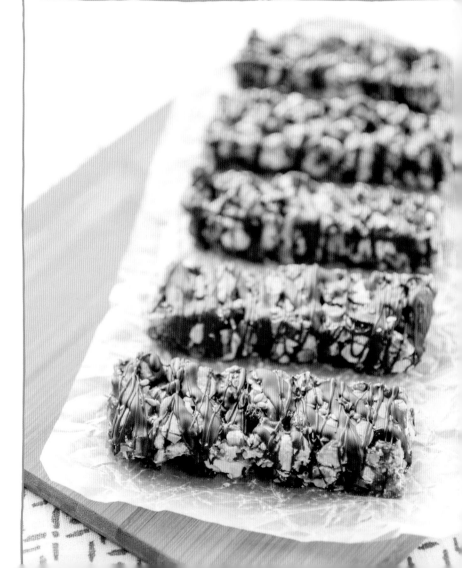

(1) Grease a large bowl, a 9 x 13-inch (23 x 33 cm) baking sheet or pan, a wooden spoon or rubber spatula, and the bottom of a drinking glass. Set aside.

(2) Add the nuts and dried fruit to the bowl, breaking apart clumps of fruit to distribute evenly throughout the mix. Add the flaxseeds. Stir to combine and set aside.

(3) In 1½- or 2-quart (1.5 or 2 L) saucepan over medium-high heat, combine the honey, maple syrup, salt, and vanilla. Cook, stirring frequently, until the mixture reaches 260°F (127°C, hard ball stage) on a candy thermometer.

(4) Immediately pour over the nut mixture and stir until evenly coated. Quickly transfer to the baking sheet or pan, using lightly greased hands to spread the mixture evenly, pressing to close in any holes. Use the bottom of the drinking glass to tap and compact the mixture in the pan.

(5) Let cool for 20 minutes (the pan should still be slightly warm). Invert the pan onto a cutting board and tap until the mixture falls out in one piece. Cut into 20 bars. (If they cool too much and become too hard or brittle to cut easily, put in a warm oven for 1 to 2 minutes to soften; then proceed with cutting.)

(6) For a chocolate drizzle, melt the chocolate chips in the top of a double boiler. Drizzle over the granola bars, if desired.

(7) Allow to cool completely before transferring to an airtight storage container with parchment paper between layers or in individual zipper-sealed plastic bags. Store at room temperature for up to 1 week. Refrigerate or freeze them to extend storage or if you prefer firmer, less sticky bars.

NOTE  You can use raw nuts and roast them yourself. Preheat the oven to 350°F (180°C, or gas mark 4). Spread the nuts on a large-size baking sheet and bake for 10 minutes or until lightly toasted and fragrant.

## FOR GLAZE:

1½ cups (180 g) powdered sugar

3 to 4 tablespoons (45 to 60 ml) milk

## FOR DOUGHNUTS:

1 cup (192 g) potato starch

½ cup (60 g) tapioca starch

½ cup (56 g) blanched almond flour

⅓ cup (64 g) cane sugar

¼ cup (45 g) potato flour

1 tablespoon (8 g) baking powder (page 20)

½ teaspoon sea salt

¼ cup (55 g) cooking fat, melted

2 large eggs, separated

⅔ cup (160 ml) milk

¼ cup (60 g) plain whole milk yogurt

2 teaspoons vanilla extract

Lard or palm oil, for frying

Pinch of cream of tartar

Yield: 8 to 10 doughnuts

# CAKE DOUGHNUTS
## (PLAIN, CHOCOLATE, OR PUMPKIN SPICE)

When I was creating recipes for this book, our friends were gracious taste testers. My husband and his friend Jeff were watching college football when I was working on this doughnut recipe. Jeff proclaimed that they were better than freshly made "Krispy Kreme" doughnuts. Mission accomplished!

① To make the glaze: Place the sugar in a bowl and slowly stir in the milk, making a smooth, pourable glaze. Set the glaze aside until the doughnuts are slightly cool.

② To make the doughnuts: In the bowl of a stand mixer fitted with the paddle attachment, combine the potato starch, tapioca starch, almond flour, sugar, potato flour, baking powder, and salt, blending on low speed. Add the fat and blend on medium-low. The mixture should resemble coarse sand.

③ In a separate bowl, combine the egg yolks, milk, yogurt, and vanilla. With the mixer running, slowly pour the wet ingredients into the dry. Scrape down the sides and mix for 30 seconds. The batter should be smooth, thick, and spoonable. Let it rest for 15 minutes.

④ Cut ten 4-inch (10 cm) squares of parchment paper and lightly grease. Set aside. Line a plate with paper towels.

(5) Heat approximately 2 inches (5 cm) of lard or palm oil in a heavy-bottomed pot to 350°F (180°C).

(6) Whisk the egg whites with a pinch of cream of tartar until soft peaks form and then fold into the rested batter.

(7) Fill a piping bag fitted with a ⅓-inch (8 mm) round tip. Pipe a 3-inch (7.5 cm)-diameter ring onto each square of parchment. Carefully place one in the oil, parchment side up (yes, leave the parchment paper attached!). Using tongs, remove the parchment paper when it comes loose. Cook each doughnut for 1 to 2 minutes on each side or until light golden brown.

(8) Remove the doughnut with a slotted spoon and drain on the paper towel–lined plate. Let cool slightly, arrange the doughnuts on a cooling rack (place a pan underneath to collect drips), and drizzle with the reserved glaze when slightly cool.

(9) *Drop Doughnut Holes:* Drop dough by rounded tablespoons (15 g) directly into the oil and fry for about 45 seconds per side or until light golden brown.

(10) *Chocolate Variation:* Add ¼ cup (20 g) cocoa powder, ½ teaspoon baking soda, and an extra 2 tablespoons (24 g) cane sugar to the dry ingredients.

(11) *Pumpkin Variation:* Use pumpkin puree in place of the yogurt and add 2 teaspoons of pumpkin pie spice.

# Chapter 5:

# APPETIZERS, SIDES, AND SNACKS

I JUST LOVE the little extras in life, especially when it comes to eating! I enjoy being able to taste small bites of many different flavors: appetizers at the beginning of the meal with a glass of wine, fun side dishes to the main course while around the dinner table, and snacks later on while relaxing with friends. No matter what the occasion, those extras are always the most exciting.

The biggest problem most people encounter when they first start out eating grain-free, however, isn't what to serve as a main dish—they get hung up on the little plates surrounding it. These appetizers, sides, and snacks are typically either filled with grains or completely boring.

In this chapter, I've put together an amazing collection of recipes for you, foods that you wouldn't be able to have anywhere else because they'd contain grains. Too often even foods that "seem" to be healthy options, such as a creamy spinach and artichoke dip, can still contain hidden grains. (And if you can't get a definitive answer from the party host or restaurant whether a food is made with grains, then when in doubt, go without.)

Appetizers represent the beginning of the evening, and the excitement and anticipation of good food and great company to come. But you don't have to limit your appetizers to boring crudité or a cheese platter. With traditionally grain-laden foods transformed into grain-free treats such as Fried Calamari (page 74), Spinach and Artichoke Dip (page 70), and Egg Rolls (page 80), you can tempt your guests with a variety of sneakily healthy options.

Side dishes not only add a variety of vitamins, minerals, and nutrients to a healthy diet, but they also more importantly liven up the dinner table with color and flavor. Of course, your meals should regularly include a colorful selection of vegetable side dishes. Whether vegetables are steamed, roasted, or pureed, the sky is the limit when it comes to how to prepare them. I've included family-favorite side dishes that you've likely served regularly with meals. Mac-a-Phony and Cheese (page 90), Green Bean Casserole (page 86) and Classic Dressing/Stuffing (page 91) can still be your go-to side dishes, even if you are grain-free!

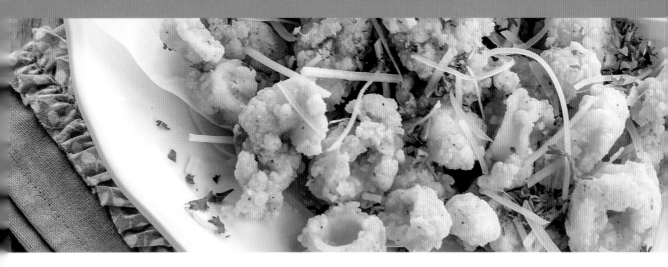

Finally, although when you eat a diet full of healthy fat and proteins, you won't feel the need to snack in between meals, there are still times when the demands of the day or occasion mean you might need to eat a little bit more before or after your next meal. For those times when you just gotta have a crunchy snack from your past, no worries, I've got you covered! Crackers (pages 81 and 83) and Tortilla Chips (page 82) are no longer off-limits. One of our favorite Saturday movie-night snacks are giant nacho platters piled high with tortilla chips and topped with Cheese Sauce (page 42), ground beef, shredded lettuce, sliced jalapeños, salsa, and tons of guacamole.

Still, just as doing a kitchen overhaul will keep you from sabotaging your health by accidentally eating grain-filled foods, keeping a few quick and easy grain-free snacks on hand will prevent you from succumbing to a serious case of the munchies. Chances are, you probably have a few of these already in your kitchen, and they don't require any preparation at all:

- Cans of tuna/sardines
- Beef jerky
- Nuts
- Fresh fruit
- Dried fruit
- Uncured cold cuts
- Pickles
- Olives
- Dark chocolate
- Trail mix

Whether you're looking to set a festive mood, enhance a hearty meal, or nibble at night, these recipes will make your meal planning more exciting and keep you from feeling deprived.

## FOR SAUCE:

⅓ cup (80 ml) hot pepper sauce (such as Frank's RedHot or Tabasco)

¼ cup (55 g) butter or ghee

1 teaspoon apple cider vinegar

1 clove of garlic, pressed or minced

Splash of Worcestershire sauce

## FOR WINGS:

1 cup (115 g) Breading Mix (page 35)

½ teaspoon garlic powder

½ teaspoon sea salt

¼ teaspoon cayenne pepper

12 whole chicken wings, separated into 12 drumettes and 12 wingettes

Optional: Lard or palm oil, for frying

YIELD: 4 SERVINGS

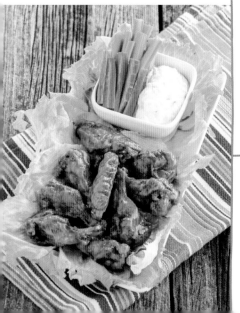

# BUFFALO WINGS

Restaurant-style buffalo chicken wings can be prepared in the comfort of your own home with a few simple ingredients and no risk of grain or gluten cross-contamination.

① To make the sauce: In a small-size saucepan over medium heat, combine the hot sauce, butter, vinegar, garlic, and Worcestershire sauce. Bring to a simmer while whisking. As soon as the liquid begins to bubble, remove from the heat and set aside.

② To make the wings: Place the breading mix, garlic powder, salt, and pepper into a resalable plastic bag and shake to mix. Add the chicken wings, seal, and toss until the wings are lightly coated with the breading mixture. Place on wax paper–lined plate(s) and refrigerate for at least 1 hour.

③ *Baked Wings:* Preheat the oven to 400°F (200°C, or gas mark 6). Line a baking sheet with parchment paper. Bake the wings until they are no longer pink in the center and are crispy on the outside, about 45 minutes. Turn the wings over halfway during baking so they cook evenly. Remove from the oven and toss with the sauce just before serving.

④ *Deep-Fried Wings:* Heat the oil in a deep-fryer or large heavy-bottomed pot to 350°F (180°C). Fry the wings in batches until crispy, about 15 minutes. Drain on a paper towel–lined plate and toss with the sauce just before serving.

NOTE   For "naked" wings, omit the breading and proceed with either the baked or the deep-fried version of this recipe.

# TURKEY, BACON, AND SWISS LETTUCE WRAPS

These wraps are the perfect cool and crisp starter to a meal or a quick snack to use up leftover holiday turkey or chicken. We especially enjoy them made with fresh garden tomatoes and a bowl of soup.

1 large-size tomato, coarsely chopped

6 slices of nitrate-free bacon, cooked and crumbled

1 cup (140 g) shredded cooked turkey (or chicken)

1 cup (110 g) shredded Swiss cheese

1 cup (225 g) mayonnaise

2 tablespoons (8 g) chopped fresh parsley

Sea salt and black pepper, to taste

4 to 8 Bibb or butter crunch lettuce leaves

YIELD: 4 SERVINGS

(1) In a medium bowl, combine the tomato, bacon, turkey, cheese, mayonnaise, and parsley and mix well. Season with the salt and pepper.

(2) Divide the mixture among the lettuce leaves and then roll them up like a burrito. Serve immediately.

NOTE  The mixture can be made up to 3 days ahead and filled into lettuce leaves just before serving.

# SPINACH AND ARTICHOKE DIP

Who can deny the popularity—or deliciousness—of artichokes and spinach blended with cheeses? The problem is that most often it's sneakily filled with grains as thickeners and served with crackers and tortilla chips that can easily contaminate the whole bowl! Next time you're invited to a party, bring this hot, flavorful dip with Breadsticks (page 45), Everything Crackers (page 81), Tortilla Chips (page 82), or cut veggies.

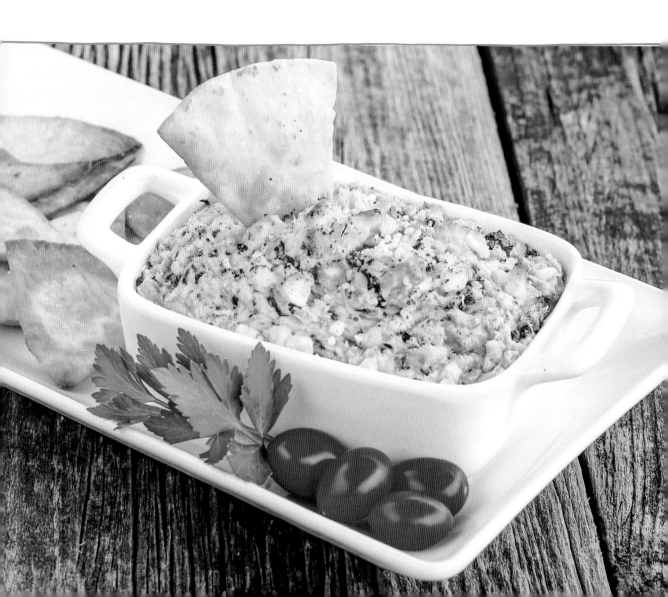

① Preheat the oven to 350°F (180°C, or gas mark 4).

② In a large skillet over medium heat, melt the butter. Add the spinach, artichokes, garlic, pepper, and nutmeg and sauté for 2 minutes or until everything is heated through and the garlic is fragrant.

③ Remove the skillet from the heat and stir in the cream cheese and mayonnaise until combined and melted.

④ In a separate bowl, combine the egg and cream. Add the mozzarella, feta, and ½ cup (50 g) of the Parmesan cheese. Add the cheese mixture to the skillet and season with salt and pepper.

⑤ Transfer the dip to a medium-size (approximately 1½-quart, or 1.5 L) ovenproof casserole dish and top with the remaining ¼ cup (25 g) Parmesan cheese.

⑥ Bake for 15 minutes or until hot and bubbly.

2 tablespoons (28 g) butter

One bag (10 ounces, or 280 g) frozen spinach, thawed and squeezed of excess liquid

1 can (14 ounces, or 390 g) artichoke hearts in brine, drained and chopped

2 cloves of garlic, minced or pressed

Pinch of crushed red pepper

Pinch of ground nutmeg

4 ounces (115 g) cream cheese

¼ cup (60 g) mayonnaise

1 large egg, beaten

⅓ cup (80 ml) heavy cream

1 cup (115 g) shredded mozzarella cheese

½ cup (75 g) crumbled feta cheese

¾ cup (75 g) Parmesan cheese, divided

Sea salt and black pepper, to taste

YIELD: 8 TO 10 SERVINGS

NOTES   The dip can be made ahead of time, stored in the refrigerator, and baked just before serving. Additionally, the unbaked dip can be frozen; allow it to thaw in the refrigerator prior to baking for best results.

Ten ounces (280 g) of fresh spinach can be used in place of frozen. Extend the sauté time to cook the fresh spinach through (until wilted).

Two cups (600 g) of frozen artichoke hearts can be used in place of canned. Use additional sea salt to season because they will not be brined.

# BACON-WRAPPED JALAPEÑO POPPERS WITH RANCH DIP

These poppers are *unbelievably* good! The crunchy-crispy exterior hides a creamy, rich filling that is nearly outdone by the flavorful ranch dip.

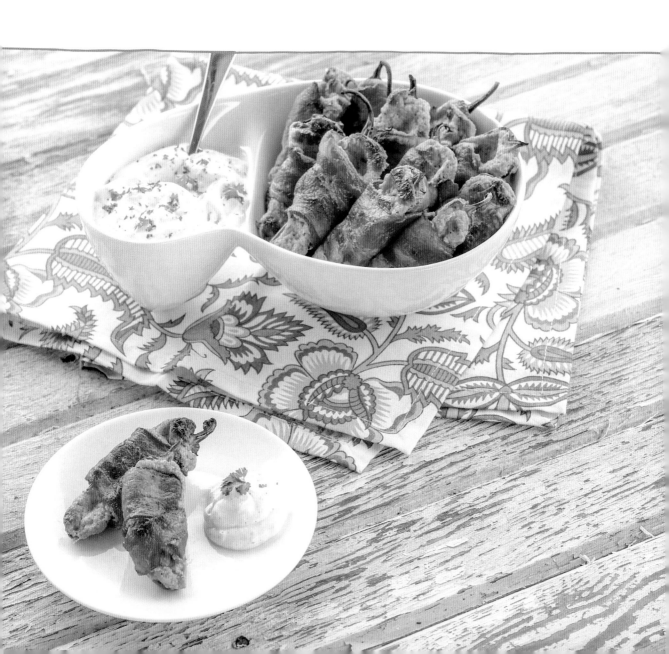

① Preheat the oven to 400°F (200°C, or gas mark 6).

② To make the ranch dip: In a small bowl, combine the mayonnaise, sour cream, and spices and mix well. Chill in the fridge until ready to serve.

③ To make the poppers: Arrange the bacon on a cookie sheet that has sides and par-bake for 15 minutes. Remove from the oven and set aside.

④ Meanwhile, in a medium-size bowl, whip together the cream cheese and seasonings using a hand or stand mixer. Add the Cheddar cheese.

⑤ Halve the peppers lengthwise and remove the seeds and membranes. Fill each half with the cream cheese mixture, wrap with half a slice of bacon, and secure with a toothpick.

⑥ Arrange the jalapeño poppers on a broiler tray and bake for 10 minutes. Then turn the broiler on high and broil for approximately 5 minutes until the bacon is crisp.

⑦ Remove from the oven and allow to cool before eating. Serve with the ranch dip, if desired.

**FOR RANCH DIP:**

¼ cup (60 g) mayonnaise

¼ cup (60 g) sour cream

¼ teaspoon dried parsley

¼ teaspoon dried chives

¼ teaspoon onion powder

⅛ teaspoon dried dill weed

⅛ teaspoon garlic powder or granulated garlic

⅛ teaspoon finely ground sea salt

⅛ teaspoon finely ground black pepper

**FOR POPPERS:**

12 slices of nitrate-free bacon, cut in half crosswise

8 ounces (225 g) cream cheese, softened

¼ teaspoon chili powder

¼ teaspoon ground cumin

¼ teaspoon sea salt

⅛ teaspoon garlic powder

⅛ teaspoon onion powder

⅛ teaspoon dried oregano

⅛ teaspoon paprika

⅛ teaspoon ground black pepper

1 cup (115 g) shredded Cheddar cheese

12 medium-large jalapeño peppers (Wear gloves when handling.)

**YIELD: 24 JALAPEÑO POPPERS**

NOTES  For extra-spicy poppers, add ¼ teaspoon red pepper flakes to the cheese mixture and/or use a pepper Jack cheese in place of the Cheddar cheese.

Depending on the size of the jalapeños, you may have extra cheese mixture left over. Use it as a spread on Everything Crackers (page 81).

1 cup (120 g) tapioca starch

½ cup (56 g) blanched
almond flour

½ cup (50 g) grated Parmesan
cheese, plus shredded for
serving

Pinch of black pepper

1 pound (454 g) calamari,
cleaned and sliced
into approximately ½-inch
(1.3 cm)-thick rings

3 egg whites, beaten

Lard or palm oil, for frying

Sea salt, to taste

Chopped fresh parsley

YIELD: 4 SERVINGS

# FRIED CALAMARI

Although fried calamari is often eaten as bar food, my favorite way to enjoy it is atop a Caesar salad—try it and you'll be hooked, too. Double-dredging the calamari in the breading mixture makes it extra crispy, which is the perfect replacement for croutons. Serve calamari with lemon slices and tomato sauce for dipping.

① In a medium-size bowl, combine the starch, flour, Parmesan cheese, and pepper, using a whisk to break up any lumps. Mix well.

② Dredge the calamari in the dry ingredients, dip into the egg whites, and dip back into the dry mix.

③ In a Dutch oven or other heavy-bottomed 5-quart (4.7 L) pot, heat approximately 2 inches (5 cm) of fat to 300°F (150°C). Line a plate with paper towels.

④ Working in small batches, fry the rings for 1 minute. (They will be crispy and light in color.) Drain on the paper towel–lined plate and season lightly with salt.

⑤ Garnish with the parsley and shredded Parmesan cheese.

NOTES   Fried calamari can be reheated by quickly dipping back into hot oil for 10 seconds. A double fry is also great if you want an extra crispy breading.

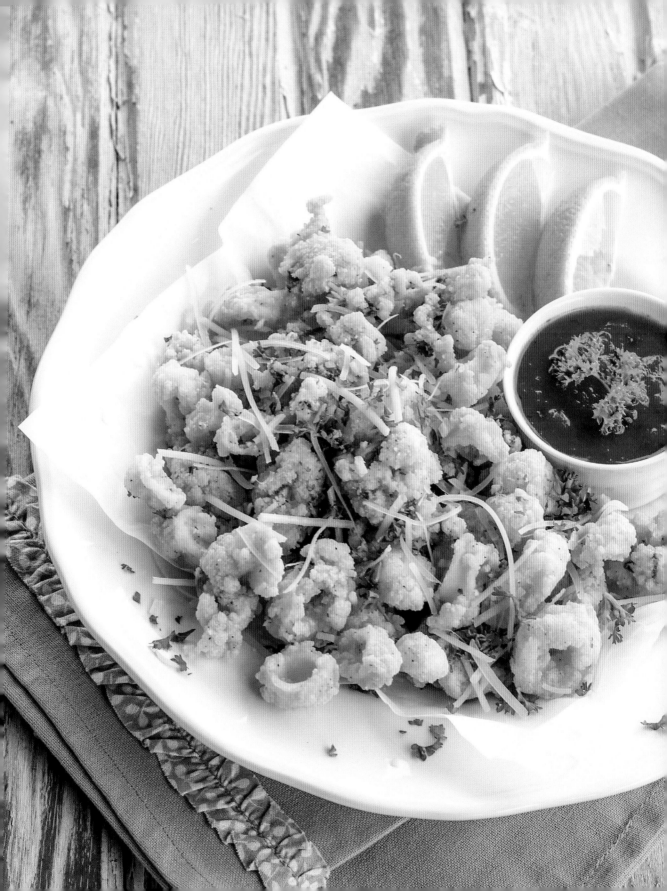

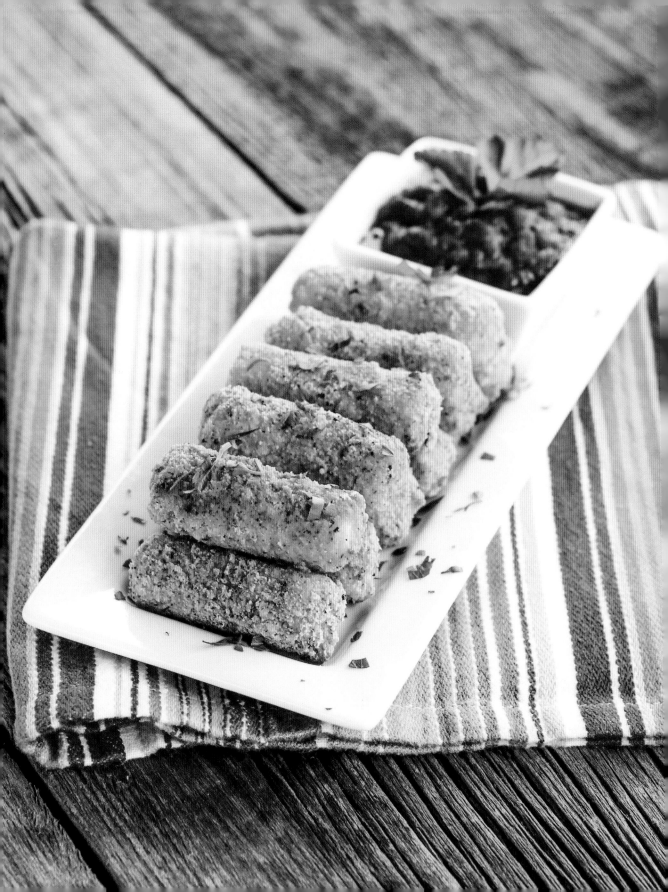

# MOZZARELLA CHEESE STICKS

There are two secrets to making perfect, grain-free mozzarella cheese sticks: making sure the layers of breading completely coat the cheese sticks and freezing them before frying. It's a little extra work, but it's worth it when you taste them. Serve them with Ranch Dip (page 73) or tomato sauce.

½ cup (56 g) blanched almond flour

½ cup (60 g) tapioca starch

¼ cup (25 g) grated Parmesan cheese

¾ teaspoon garlic powder

¾ teaspoon onion powder

¾ teaspoon sea salt

¾ teaspoon Italian seasoning

¼ teaspoon white pepper

12 mozzarella string cheese sticks (1 ounce, or 28 g each)

2 large eggs, beaten

Lard or palm oil, for frying

YIELD: 24 CHEESE STICKS

① In a food processor, combine the flour, starch, Parmesan, and seasonings and process until well combined.

② Cut each string cheese stick in half, creating 2 shorter sticks. Roll each stick in the dry ingredients, then into the eggs, then into the dry, then back into the eggs, and finally back into the dry (dry-egg-dry-egg-dry).

③ Make sure each stick is completely coated and the breading is sealed. Arrange them on a wax paper–lined plate(s) and freeze for at least 2 hours.

④ In a Dutch oven or other large heavy-bottomed pot, heat approximately 2 inches (5 cm) of fat to 350°F (180°C). Line a plate with paper towels. Fry the frozen cheese sticks just until the cheese starts to leak out, about 2 to 3 minutes.

⑤ Allow them to drain on a paper towel–lined plate and cool slightly before eating.

## SOUTHWEST QUESADILLAS

2 tablespoons (28 ml) melted cooking fat, divided

1 small onion, sliced

½ of a green bell pepper, sliced

Sea salt, to taste

4 Tortillas (page 41)

8 ounces (225 g) cooked steak, cut into ¼-inch (6 mm)-thick pieces, or shredded cooked chicken

1 cup (115 g) shredded Cheddar cheese

Optional toppings: salsa, sour cream, guacamole, and fresh cilantro

YIELD: 4 SERVINGS

Quesadillas are a great way to use leftover cooked meat or chicken. Serve as a snack, an appetizer, or an easy dinner when time is short. Serve with sour cream, guacamole, and lots of salsa.

① Heat 2 teaspoons (10 ml) of the fat in a 10-inch (25 cm) skillet over medium heat. Add the onion and pepper and cook, stirring, until softened, about 5 to 10 minutes. Season the mixture with salt and transfer to a bowl.

② Brush 1 side of each tortilla with the remaining 4 teaspoons (20 ml) fat. Place 1 tortilla, oil-side down, in the same skillet; sprinkle with half the steak, half the onion mixture, and ½ cup (58 g) of the cheese. Place a second tortilla, oil-side up, on top of the cheese, pressing down with a spatula to seal.

③ Cook the quesadilla until the cheese melts and the tortillas are browned, about 3 to 4 minutes per side. Remove the quesadilla from the skillet and cut into wedges. Repeat with the remaining ingredients for a second quesadilla.

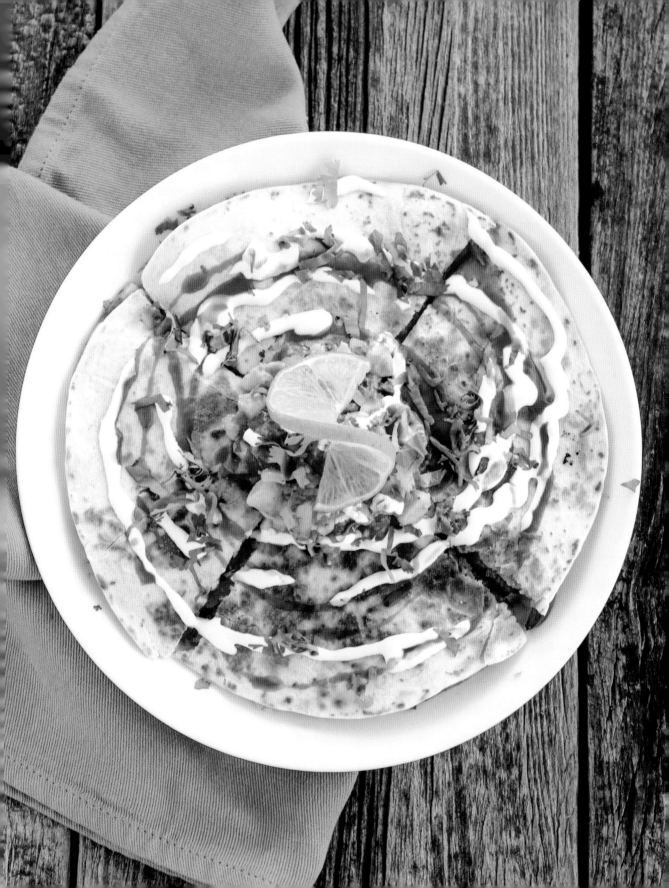

- 1 pound (455 g) ground pork, chicken, or turkey
- 1 small onion, chopped
- 2 cloves of garlic, pressed or minced
- 1 teaspoon grated ginger
- ¼ cup (60 ml) coconut aminos
- 2 carrots, grated
- 4 cups (300 g) shredded napa cabbage, approximately ½ of a medium head
- Sea salt and black pepper, to taste
- 14 to 16 tapioca sheets (banh trang)
- Lard or palm oil, for frying
- Optional: hot sauce or duck sauce, for dipping

YIELD: 14 TO 16 EGG ROLLS

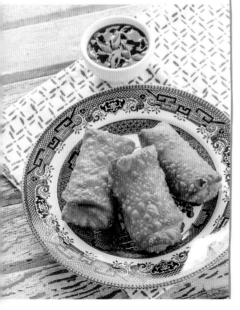

# EGG ROLLS

The key to making grain-free egg rolls is wrapper sheets made of tapioca starch. Tapioca sheets (banh trang) can be found at most Asian stores. Be sure to verify that there is no rice or wheat in the ingredients list.

① In a large skillet over medium heat, cook the pork, breaking it up into small pieces. Add the onion, garlic, ginger, and coconut aminos and cook for 2 minutes or until the pork is no longer pink.

② Quickly stir in the carrots and cabbage, cooking just until they are wilted and water has been released, about 3 minutes. Season with the salt and pepper.

③ Transfer the mixture to a colander set over a bowl to drain off any excess liquid and place in the fridge to cool.

④ Fill a pie plate, or other shallow container that is large enough to hold the tapioca sheets, with warm water. Submerge one sheet in the water for 2 to 3 minutes or until soft.

⑤ Lay the softened tapioca sheet on a flat work surface. Place approximately ¼ cup (55 g) of the filling just below the center of the circle and shape into a log, leaving about 1 inch (2.5 cm) free along the edges. Fold the bottom up over the filling and roll up just enough to tuck the end under. Fold each side over toward the center and continue rolling up (forward) to the far end of the circle. Place the egg rolls on a plate or tray, being careful that they do not touch each other.

⑥ In a Dutch oven or other large-size heavy-bottomed pot, heat 2 to 3 inches (5 to 7.5 cm) of fat to 350°F (180°C). Line a plate with paper towels.

⑦ Deep fry the egg rolls for 3 to 5 minutes or until brown. Remove and drain on the paper towel–lined plate. Serve with hot sauce or duck sauce, if desired.

# EVERYTHING CRACKERS

Making grain-free crackers is quick, easy, and fun. They can be made with various toppings: onion, garlic, sesame seeds, poppy seeds, or everything!

**FOR TOPPING:**

1 teaspoon sesame seeds

½ teaspoon poppy seeds

¼ teaspoon garlic powder

¼ teaspoon onion powder

**FOR CRACKERS:**

½ cup (56 g) blanched almond flour

½ cup (60 g) tapioca starch

½ teaspoon garlic powder

½ teaspoon onion powder

½ teaspoon sea salt

¼ teaspoon white pepper

½ cup (120 ml) water

### Yield: 4 servings

① Preheat the oven to 400°F (200°C, or gas mark 6) and line a baking sheet with parchment paper.

② To make the topping: Combine all the topping ingredients in a small bowl and set aside.

③ To make the crackers: In a medium-size bowl, combine the flour, starch, powders, salt, and pepper. Add the water and stir. The mixture will resemble a thin pancake batter.

④ Pour the batter onto the prepared baking sheet and spread thin.

⑤ Bake for 5 minutes, remove from the oven, and sprinkle with the topping. Return to the oven and bake for an additional 25 minutes or until crispy.

⑥ Remove from the oven and cut or break into desired cracker-size squares. Transfer the crackers and parchment to a cooling rack. Store in an airtight container or sealed bag for several weeks.

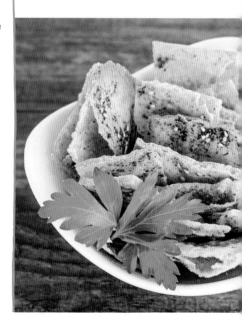

**4 Tortillas (page 41)**

**Lard or palm oil, for frying**

**Sea salt**

Yield: 32 Tortilla chips

# TORTILLA CHIPS

Yes, you *can* have tortilla chips even though you're eating grain-free! Serve these with salsa, guacamole, Cheese Sauce (page 42), or Spinach and Artichoke Dip (page 70).

(1) Cut each tortilla into 8 wedges and set aside.

(2) In a low-sided skillet (preferably cast iron), heat ½ to ¾ inch (1.3 to 2 cm) of fat over medium-high heat to approximately 350°F (180°C). Line a plate with paper towels.

(3) Fry the tortilla wedges in a single layer, turning so that both sides are lightly brown, 1 to 2 minutes per side. Remove the crispy chips from the oil and place on a paper towel–lined plate. Season with salt.

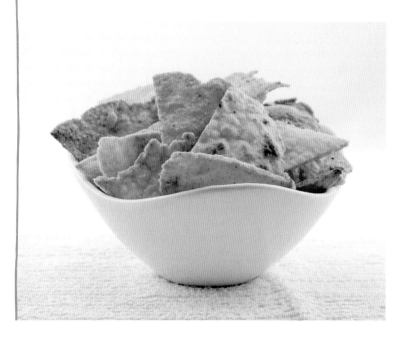

# CHEESE "IT" CRACKERS

These cheesy crackers are so quick and easy to make, you'll almost think you're eating the store-bought version!

① Preheat the oven to 400°F (200°C, or gas mark 6).

② In a food processor, combine all the ingredients and process until a smooth dough is formed.

③ Roll out the dough between 2 pieces of parchment paper into an 8 x 12-inch (20 by 30 cm) rectangle. Transfer the parchment and dough to a baking sheet and remove the top layer.

④ Use a pizza cuter or knife to score the dough into 1-inch (2.5 cm) squares (the pieces will not be separated yet).

⑤ Bake for 10 minutes and then remove from the oven and recut along the same lines as before baking. Return to the oven and bake for an additional 10 to 15 minutes or until the pieces are crispy.

⑥ Carefully transfer the crackers on the parchment onto a cooling rack and allow to cool before breaking on the scored lines into individual crackers. The crackers can be stored in an airtight container for several weeks.

2 cups (225 g) shredded Cheddar cheese

⅓ cup (37 g) blanched almond flour

⅓ cup (40 g) tapioca starch

3 tablespoons (42 g) butter, softened

3 tablespoons (45 ml) water

1 teaspoon coconut sugar

½ teaspoon garlic powder

½ teaspoon onion powder

¼ teaspoon baking powder (page 20)

¼ teaspoon sea salt

¼ teaspoon white pepper

⅛ teaspoon arrowroot starch

Pinch of crushed red pepper

## YIELD: 4 SERVINGS

1½ cups (173 g) Breading Mix
(page 34), divided

1 large egg, separated

⅓ cup (80 ml) gluten-free
beer or club soda, chilled

1 tablespoon (14 g) cooking
fat, melted

Sea salt, to taste

2 large-size Vidalia or other
sweet onions, sliced into
rings

Lard or palm oil, for frying

Yield: 4 servings

# BEER BATTER ONION RINGS

Impress your family with homemade onion rings that taste just as good as the ones from the local diner, only these are grain-free. Serve with a side of ketchup.

① Set aside ½ cup (58 g) of the breading mix for dusting the onion rings. In a separate large-size bowl, whisk the egg yolk and then add the beer and fat. Slowly add the remaining 1 cup (115 g) breading mix and mix well. Allow the mixture to stand for 15 minutes.

② In a Dutch oven or other large-size heavy-bottomed pot, heat 2 to 3 inches (5 to 7.5 cm) of fat to 350°F (180°C). Line a plate with paper towels.

③ In a small-size bowl with a hand mixer or whisk, stiffly beat the egg white. Gently fold into the batter.

④ Dust each onion ring with the reserved breading mix and then dip into the batter. Deep fry the battered rings, several at a time, for 2 to 3 minutes or until golden brown. Drain on the paper towel–lined plate, season with salt, and serve.

# CREAMED SPINACH

I've been making this creamed spinach recipe since
I was in college, when I found out that many versions
of creamed spinach sneakily use flour as a thickener in
the sauce. It tastes like a complicated restaurant dish,
but is very easy.

2 tablespoons (28 g)
    cooking fat

1 medium-size onion, finely
    chopped

2 cloves of garlic, pressed
    or minced

One bag (10 ounces, or 280 g)
    baby spinach or baby kale

Pinch of crushed red pepper

Sea salt and black pepper,
    to taste

⅓ cup (80 ml) heavy cream

¼ cup (25 g) grated Parmesan
    cheese

## YIELD: 4 SERVINGS

① In a large skillet over medium heat, melt the fat. Add the onion
and garlic and sauté until soft, about 5 minutes. Add the spinach
and toss with tongs, adding a little more fat, if needed. Cook the
spinach just until wilted.

② Season with red pepper, salt, and black pepper. Reduce the heat
to medium-low and add the cream and Parmesan cheese. Stir well.

③ Allow to simmer until slightly reduced and thickened, about
1 to 2 minutes more.

½ cup (112 g) cooking fat, divided

1 small onion, finely chopped

1 pound (455 g) button mushrooms, cleaned and chopped

2 teaspoons sea salt, divided

½ teaspoon ground black pepper, divided

1½ pounds (680 g) fresh green beans, trimmed and cut into 2-inch (5 cm) pieces

¼ cup (48 g) potato starch

2 cups (475 ml) milk

Pinch of cayenne pepper

Pinch of grated nutmeg

1 cup (100 g) grated Parmesan cheese, divided

¼ cup (30 g) bread crumbs (page 39)

1 large onion, thinly sliced

## Yield: 6 to 8 servings

# GREEN BEAN CASSEROLE

It's the dish everyone's expecting on the holiday table, but it's simple enough to make any day. This version isn't made with canned, grain-filled condensed soups or grain-coated crispy canned onions; it's healthy, real food made from scratch. For a special treat, top with Beer Batter Onion Rings (page 84).

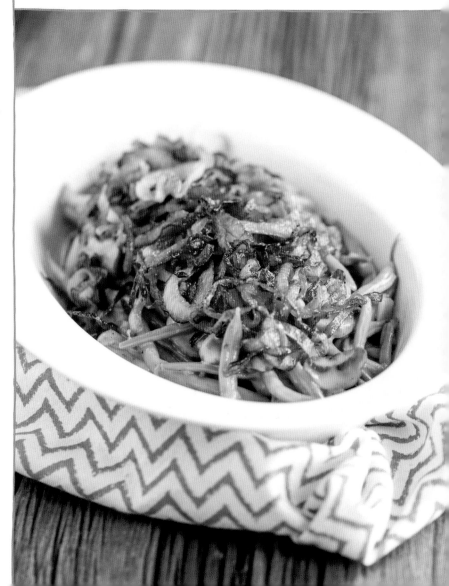

①  Preheat the oven to 350°F (180°C, or gas mark 4). Butter a 9 x 13-inch (23 x 33 cm) baking dish.

②  In a large skillet over medium heat, melt 2 tablespoons (28 g) of the fat. Add the onion and sauté until it begins to soften, about 4 minutes. Add the mushrooms and cook until softened and most of the liquid has evaporated, about 8 minutes. Season with 1 teaspoon of the salt and ¼ teaspoon of the pepper. Set aside to cool.

③  Prepare an ice bath by filling a large bowl with ice and water; set aside. Bring a large saucepan of water to a boil. Add the green beans and cook until bright green and just tender, about 3 to 5 minutes. Drain and transfer to the ice bath to stop the cooking. When cooled, drain and toss the beans with the mushroom mixture.

④  Melt ¼ cup (55 g) of the fat in a medium saucepan over medium-low heat. Add the potato starch and whisk constantly to break up any lumps. Pour in the milk and continue whisking until the mixture has thickened, about 3 minutes. Stir in the cayenne, nutmeg, and remaining 1 teaspoon salt and ¼ teaspoon pepper. Remove from the heat and let cool to room temperature, stirring occasionally. Pour over the beans and toss to combine.

⑤  Spread half the green bean mixture over the bottom of the prepared baking dish. Sprinkle on ½ cup (50 g) of the grated Parmesan and spread with the remaining green beans. Combine the remaining ½ cup (50 g) Parmesan and the bread crumbs and sprinkle over the casserole. Cover with foil.

⑥  In a medium skillet over medium-high heat, sauté the sliced onions in the remaining 2 tablespoons (28 g) of fat until soft, about 3 to 5 minutes. Set aside until ready to serve.

⑦  Bake the casserole, covered, until the mixture is bubbly and heated through, about 10 minutes. Turn the oven to broil, uncover, and broil approximately 8 inches (20 cm) from the heating element, with the oven door slightly ajar, about 30 seconds. Sprinkle the reserved fried onions over the top and serve immediately.

NOTE   The casserole can be made up to 2 days ahead of time and kept in the refrigerator. Baking time will increase to 30 to 45 minutes to heat through. Be mindful if your casserole dish needs to come to room temperature before baking to avoid breakage. After the casserole is heated through, broil and top with the onions as detailed above.

½ of recipe for Pasta Dough
(page 37)

Tapioca starch

1 medium head of cabbage

8 ounces (225 g) nitrate-free
bacon, chopped

1 medium onion, halved and
sliced

2 tablespoons (28 g) butter
or ghee

Sea salt and black pepper,
to taste

YIELD: 4 TO 6 SERVINGS

# FRIED CABBAGE AND NOODLES

A traditional dish of Polish and Slovak heritage, haluski is braised cabbage and egg noodles smothered in butter. Growing up, it was a staple at my grandmother's dinner table, and today it's one of my favorite comfort foods.

① Bring a large pot of salted water to a boil.

② Divide the pasta dough into 2 equal portions. Using tapioca starch as needed to avoid sticking, roll out the dough to approximately ¼ inch (6 mm) thick. Use a pizza cutter or knife to cut noodles approximately ½ x 2 inches (1.3 x 5 cm).

③ Boil the noodles for 7 minutes, drain, and rinse with cold water. Set aside.

④ Cut the head of cabbage into quarters and remove the core. Thinly slice the cabbage quarters (almost shredded).

⑤ In a large skillet over medium-high heat, cook the bacon until crisp. Reduce the heat to medium-low, add the onion, and sauté until soft, about 3 to 4 minutes. Add the cabbage and stir to lightly sauté for 1 minute. Reduce the heat to low, cover, and cook for 2 to 3 minutes or until the cabbage is very lightly cooked.

⑥ Add the noodles and butter and turn the heat up to medium-high. Allow to cook for a few minutes, stirring often but allowing some pieces to get a little browned. Season with the salt and pepper.

NOTE   If you prefer softer cabbage, extend the cooking time (before adding the noodles) for up to 10 minutes or until the cabbage is cooked to your liking.

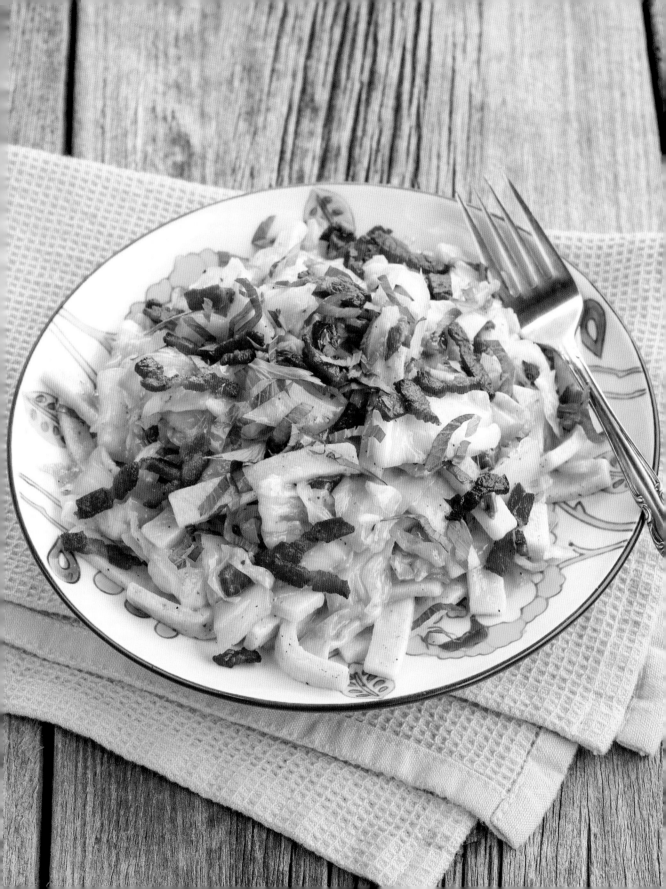

1 large head of cauliflower,
cut into small florets

1 cup (225 g) cottage cheese

½ cup (120 ml) milk

½ teaspoon dry mustard
powder

¼ teaspoon white pepper

1 teaspoon sea salt

½ teaspoon garlic powder

¼ teaspoon paprika

2 cups (225 g) shredded
Cheddar cheese

**FOR OPTIONAL TOPPINGS:**

1 cup (115 g) bread crumbs
(page 39)

1 cup (115 g) shredded
Cheddar cheese

Yield: 4 to 6 servings

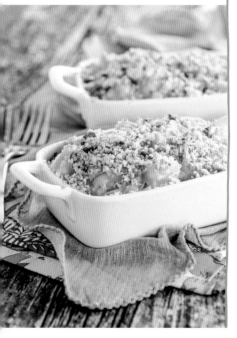

# MAC-A-PHONY AND CHEESE

This is the perfect way to get all the traditional flavors
of macaroni and cheese, only full of cauliflower instead
of pasta.

① Preheat the oven to 350°F (180°C, or gas mark 4) and butter a
3-quart (2.8 L) casserole dish.

② Fill a pot with about 1 inch (2.5 cm) of water and bring to a boil
over high heat. Place the cauliflower in a steamer insert and place
over the water. Cover with a lid and steam for about 5 minutes or
until cooked but still slightly crisp. (You do not want them soft and
falling apart, as they will continue to cook when your casserole is
baked). Transfer to a medium bowl.

③ In a blender, combine the cottage cheese, milk, and seasonings,
and blend until smooth. Transfer the blended mixture to a medium
saucepan over low heat and bring to a simmer. Add the Cheddar,
stirring continuously to melt. If the cheese sauce is not completely
smooth, return it to the blender and blend until smooth.

④ Pour the cheese sauce over the cauliflower and toss to coat.
Transfer to the prepared casserole dish. Cover with aluminum foil
and bake for 45 minutes. Remove the foil and top as desired. Bake
for an additional 5 to 10 minutes until hot and bubbly.

# CLASSIC DRESSING/STUFFING

The terms "stuffing" and "dressing" are often used interchangeably, but they do have different meanings: stuffing is cooked inside the bird; dressing is cooked on its own. This recipe is perfect whether baked in the bird or as a casserole.

① Preheat the oven to 350°F (180°C, or gas mark 4). Butter a 2-quart (2 L) baking dish.

② In a medium saucepan over medium heat, melt the fat. Add the onion and celery and sauté until softened, about 4 to 5 minutes. Add the chicken broth and simmer for 2 to 3 minutes. Remove from the heat and allow to cool.

③ Place the bread cubes in a large mixing bowl and toss with the salt, sage, pepper, thyme, and marjoram.

④ Stir the egg into the cooled onion-celery mixture and pour over the bread cubes. Mix well.

⑤ Transfer to the baking dish and bake for 45 minutes or until the top is lightly browned.

2 tablespoons (28 g) cooking fat

1 small onion, chopped

2 stalks of celery, chopped

¾ cup (175 ml) chicken broth/stock (page 93)

4 cups (200 g) cubed Sliceable Sandwich Bread (page 38)

¾ teaspoon sea salt

1 teaspoon ground sage

¼ teaspoon ground black pepper

¼ teaspoon dried thyme

¼ teaspoon dried marjoram

1 large egg, beaten

YIELD: 8 SERVINGS

NOTES  This recipe can be doubled as needed for a larger crowd. If the stuffing seems too dry, add more broth. You can also use this as stuffing in-the-bird; this recipe will fill a small (5- to 7-pound, or 2.3 to 3.2 kg) bird.

# Chapter 6:

# SOUPS AND STEWS

SOUPS ARE VERSATILE. Whether served as the starter to a meal or as the main course, soups are fitting for nearly every occasion. Similarly, stews are foolproof and practically make themselves. With just a few ingredients and a little time, you'll have a hearty, filling meal with very little effort.

However, soups and stews are notorious for sneakily containing grains and gluten, whether thickened with flour or packed with noodles. Thus, it's best to stick to homemade ones.

Not only do soups and stews taste yummy, but they are also the perfect way to incorporate nourishing bone broth into your diet. Boiling animal bones for a long period of time will release bone marrow and glycine, which can boost the immune system and help the body fend off any invading viruses and bacteria. It is also a cheap and delicious way to flood your body with vital nutrients such as collagen, gelatin, calcium, phosphorus, and magnesium that will help your body detox and start repairing damaged tissue.

Bone broth is a powerhouse of vitamins and nutrients that can heal and nourish the body from the inside. Drinking a mug of bone broth every day has been shown to help the body repair inflammation, heal a leaky gut, lessen joint pain, reverse immune disorders, and kill candida. Known as the magic elixir, bone broth was a common dish just a few decades ago and was used to add flavor to soups and sauces. Now it has been replaced with small, foil-wrapped stock bouillon cubes that simulate the taste of meat and contain none of the nutrients found in real broth. (Most of the boxed broths sold in grocery stores are as nutrient deficient as bouillon cubes; however, there are a few new brands that use bones. See Resources for my recommendations.)

Perhaps one of bone broth's greatest nutrients is gelatin, which performs a "patch and repair" service on a leaky gut. Gut hyperpermeability, or leaky gut, refers to the condition in which holes begin to appear in the intestinal lining, allowing small food particles to pass through and enter the bloodstream. As noted in chapter 1, the body will then begin to attack these food particles, and over time, this condition can lead to an autoimmune disease. Leaky gut is becoming more common and is often a symptom of irritable bowel syndrome and Crohn's disease. Many people attribute this rise to lifestyle factors such as increased stress, consumption of refined grains and sugars, and long-term use of oral contraceptives. Other research suggests that it could be due to bacterial or yeast overgrowth such as candida, which causes inflammation in the intestinal lining.

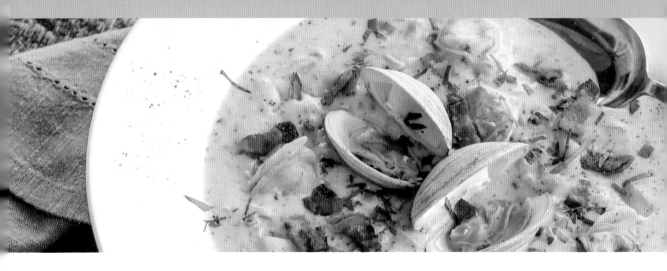

To make your own healing bone broth, you can use the bones of high quality chicken, beef, lamb, venison, pork, or fish. It is vital that you use the bones from organic, free-range animals that are fed 100 percent grass (or their natural diet equivalent) because you will be consuming the nutrients and minerals contained within these bones. You can use the broth as an ingredient in recipes such as Hearty Beef Stew (page 103), Home-Style Chicken Noodle Soup (page 107), or Italian Wedding Soup (page 109), or have a daily cup of broth as a part of your health-building routine, just like me!

# BASIC BONE BROTH

### Yield: About 12 cups (2.8 L)

**2 pounds (900 g) bones (beef, chicken, pork, or venison)**

**1 gallon (3.8 L) water**

**2 tablespoons (30 ml) raw apple cider vinegar (helps extract nutrients from the bones)**

**Sea salt, to taste**

**Optional additions: vegetables such as carrots, onions, and celery; and herbs and spices such as garlic, ginger, peppercorns, and fresh parsley stems**

① Place the bones in a slow cooker and cover with the water and vinegar. Cook on low for 36 to 48 hours. The longer the broth cooks, the more nutrients it will have. Ideally, the bones should be easily broken.

② When done, strain and season with salt. The broth will keep in the refrigerator for 7 to 10 days. After refrigeration, the fat will rise to the top where it can be easily removed. The broth can also be frozen for up to 6 months.

1 large head of broccoli

¼ cup (55 g) cooking fat, divided

1 medium onion, chopped

1 rib of celery, chopped

1 clove of garlic, pressed or minced

4 cups (950 ml) chicken broth/stock (page 93)

1 teaspoon dry mustard powder

½ teaspoon sea salt

¼ teaspoon white pepper

2 tablespoons (21 g) arrowroot or (24 g) potato starch

2 carrots, peeled and diced

4 cups (950 ml) half-and-half (or 2 cups [475 ml] milk and 2 cups [475 ml] heavy cream)

Optional: shredded Cheddar cheese

YIELD: 8 CUPS (1.9 L)

NOTE   For a thicker soup, puree 1 cup (235 ml) of the soup with an additional 1 to 2 tablespoons (11 to 21 g) arrowroot starch. Mix it back in to the soup pot until well combined and heated through.

# CREAM OF BROCCOLI SOUP

Cream of broccoli soup is best when it is homemade. On a chilly fall evening, you can be eating a filling dinner in less than an hour, from start to finish.

① Separate the broccoli florets from the stems. Divide the florets into bite-size pieces and set aside for later in this recipe (approximately 3 cups [213 g]). Discard the tough, pithy bottom stem. Coarsely chop the remaining stems (1 to 2 cups [71 to 142 g]).

② In a large pot or Dutch oven over medium heat, heat 2 tablespoons (28 g) of the fat. Sauté the broccoli stems, onion, celery, and garlic until softened, about 3 to 4 minutes.

③ Add the broth, mustard powder, salt, and pepper. Stir to incorporate.

④ Carefully transfer the cooked mixture to the blender along with the arrowroot starch and puree until completely smooth. Set aside.

⑤ To the pot, add the remaining 2 tablespoons (28 g) fat and heat over medium heat. Add the reserved broccoli florets and carrots and sauté for 2 to 3 minutes or until slightly softened.

⑥ Add the pureed mixture to the broccoli and carrots, bring to a simmer, and then reduce the heat to low, cover, and cook for 5 minutes to lightly cook the broccoli and carrots.

⑦ Remove the lid and add the half-and-half. Keep the heat on low and cook for an additional 5 minutes or until the carrots are soft. Season with additional salt and pepper to taste.

⑧ Serve bowls of creamy broccoli soup topped with shredded Cheddar cheese, if desired.

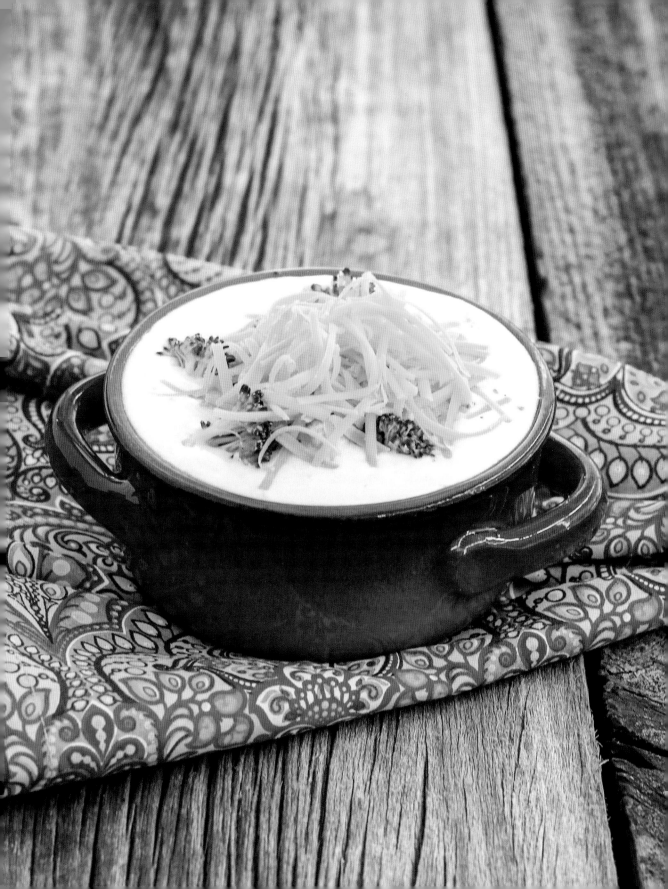

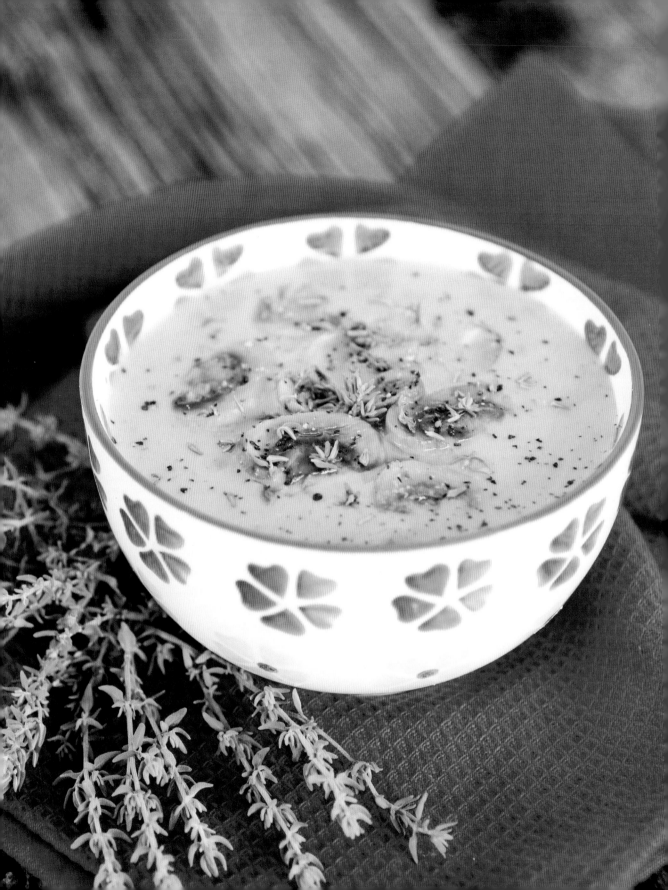

# CREAM OF MUSHROOM SOUP

Rich cream of mushroom soup beats the canned variety any day. Garnish the bowls with chopped fresh chives and thyme, if desired.

¼ cup (55 g) cooking fat

1 pound (455 g) white button mushrooms, sliced

Juice of 1 lemon wedge

1 teaspoon sea salt

1 small onion, chopped

2 cloves of garlic, pressed or minced

4 cups (950 ml) beef or chicken broth/stock (page 93)

¼ teaspoon white pepper

1 sprig of fresh thyme

1 pound (455 g) Yukon gold potatoes, peeled and cut into ½-inch (1.3 cm) cubes (about 3 cups [330 g])

4 cups (950 ml) milk

YIELD: 8 CUPS (1.9 L)

① In a 4-quart (3.8 L) pot, melt the fat over medium heat and then sauté the mushrooms with the lemon juice and salt for 5 minutes. Add the onion and garlic and continue cooking until the onion is translucent, about 2 to 3 minutes.

② Add the broth, pepper, thyme, and potatoes. Bring to a boil, then lower the heat to medium-low, cover, and simmer for 15 minutes or until the potatoes are soft and cooked through.

③ When the potatoes are cooked, remove the thyme and carefully puree approximately half of the soup in a blender until smooth. Add the pureed soup back into the pot and add the milk. Gently simmer until heated through. Season with additional salt.

- 1½ to 2 pounds (680 to 900 g) pork roast (untrimmed with bone)
- 2 tablespoons (24 g) potato starch
- 1 tablespoon (7 g) paprika
- 1 teaspoon sea salt
- 1 teaspoon garlic powder
- 1 teaspoon onion powder
- ½ teaspoon ground black pepper
- ¼ cup (55 g) cooking fat
- 2 cloves of garlic, pressed or minced
- 1 rib of celery, chopped
- 1 small onion, chopped
- 1 red, yellow, or orange bell pepper, cored, seeded, and chopped
- ½ of a green bell pepper, cored, seeded, and chopped
- 2 carrots, peeled and chopped
- 4 cups (720 g) canned chopped or diced tomatoes in juice
- 1 bay leaf
- 1 pound (455 g) russet potatoes, peeled and cubed into bite-size pieces (about 3 cups [330 g])
- Sour cream, for serving

Yield: 12 cups (2.8 L)

# HUNGARIAN GOULASH

Hungarian goulash is a perfect example of how simple ingredients can yield incredible flavor. I first had Hungarian goulash at my husband's grandmother's house, and I made sure to learn it from her. I've adapted Nan Ryczek's recipe to be grain-free so we can all enjoy its flavorful simplicity. For a little spice, substitute Hungarian wax pepper for the green bell pepper.

1) Preheat the oven to 350°F (180°C, or gas mark 4).

2) Cut the pork roast into cubes, cutting around the bone. In a large-size bowl, toss the cubes of pork and bones with the potato starch, paprika, sea salt, garlic powder, onion powder, and black pepper. (Include the bones in the goulash, as they provide flavor and healthy gelatin; you will remove them prior to serving.)

3) In a 4-quart (3.8 L) ovenproof pot with lid or a Dutch oven over medium heat, melt the fat. Brown the seasoned pork cubes and bones, about 3 to 5 minutes. Add the garlic, celery, onion, peppers, and carrots and sauté for about 5 minutes. Add the tomatoes and bay leaf, cover, transfer to the oven, and bake for 2 hours.

4) Remove the goulash from the oven, add the cubed potatoes, and bake for an additional hour (total baking time is 3 hours). Remove the bay leaf and bones. Serve bowls of goulash with a generous dollop of sour cream.

NOTES   Goulash can be started the day before, refrigerated, and then baked as directed. Or cook it in a slow cooker on low for 6 to 8 hours instead of baking, adding the potatoes 1 hour before serving.

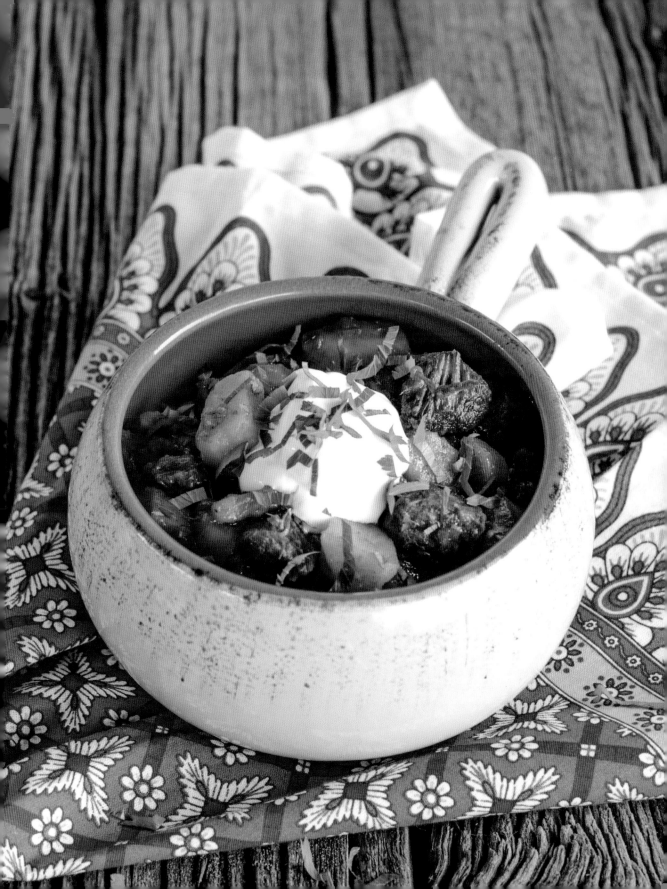

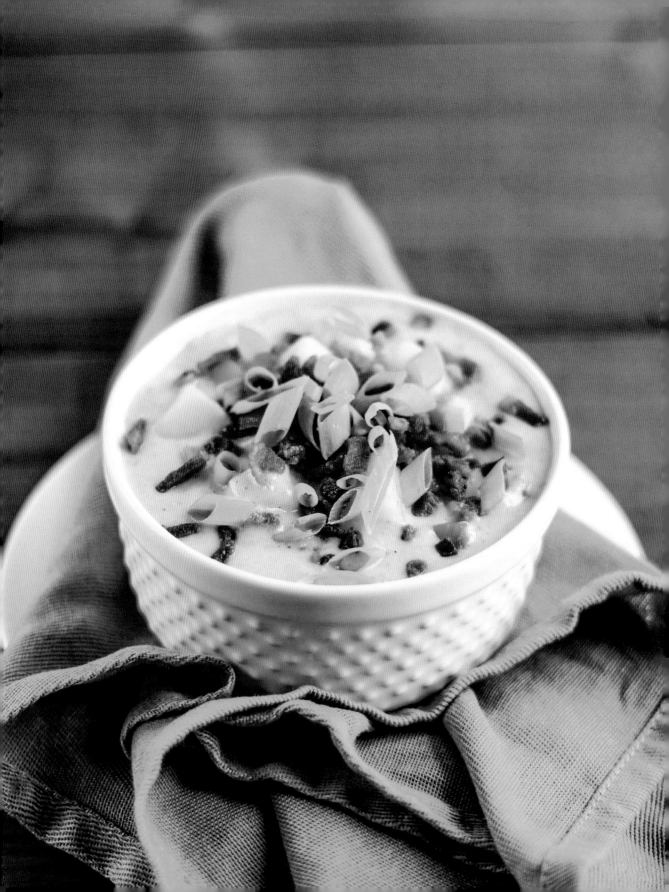

# POTATO SOUP WITH BACON AND SCALLIONS

This classic potato soup is thick, creamy, and delicious, made healthier without any flour as a thickener and with nourishing homemade bone broth.

1 In a 3-quart (2.8 L) pot over medium-high heat, sauté the bacon until crisp. Drain the bacon on a paper towel–lined plate; crumble and reserve. Pour off all but 2 tablespoons (28 ml) of the drippings and return the pot with the drippings to the heat.

2 Cook the onion, celery, carrot, and garlic in the drippings, stirring often, for about 5 minutes. Add the potatoes, stock, salt, and pepper. Bring to a boil, reduce the heat to medium-low, cover, and simmer for 15 minutes or until the potatoes are soft and cooked through.

3 Ladle approximately one-third of the cooked soup into a blender, and blend until smooth. Add it back to the pot along with the half-and-half, cream cheese, and half of the reserved bacon. Simmer, stirring, until the cream cheese melts. Season with additional sea salt and pepper.

4 Garnish individual bowls of soup with the remaining bacon and the sliced scallions.

1 pound (455 g) nitrate-free bacon, chopped

1 medium onion, chopped

2 ribs of celery, chopped

1 carrot, chopped

1 clove of garlic, pressed or minced

2 pounds (900 g) red-skinned potatoes, peeled and cut into ½-inch (1.3 cm) cubes (about 6 cups [660 g])

4 cups (950 ml) chicken broth/stock (page 93)

1 tablespoon (15 g) sea salt

¼ teaspoon white pepper

2 cups (475 ml) half-and-half (or 1 cup [235 ml] heavy cream and 1 cup [235 ml] whole milk)

4 ounces (115 g) cream cheese, softened

1 bunch of scallions, green tops sliced

YIELD: 8 CUPS (1.9 L)

2 tablespoons (28 g) cooking fat

3 large onions, sliced (any combination of yellow, white, and/or red)

4 cloves of garlic, pressed or minced

½ cup (120 ml) dry white wine

2 tablespoons (28 ml) dry sherry

2 tablespoons (21 g) arrowroot starch

2 cups (475 ml) chicken broth/stock (page 93)

2 cups (475 ml) beef broth/stock (page 93)

1 sprig of fresh thyme

Sea salt, to taste

Ground black pepper, to taste

4 slices of Sliceable Sandwich Bread (page 38), toasted

4 slices of provolone or Swiss cheese

YIELD: 4 SERVINGS

# FRENCH ONION SOUP

I've always loved a bowl of French onion soup when we go out to dinner. But even if I leave off the bread topper, the soup itself is still thickened with flour. It's dangerously deceiving for anyone avoiding grains. This recipe uses toasted Sliceable Sandwich Bread (page 38) to make it a grain-free delight at home.

① In a large Dutch oven or heavy-bottomed pot with a lid, melt the fat over medium-low heat. Add the onions and garlic, cover, and sweat for 10 minutes. Remove the lid and continue cooking the onions, stirring occasionally, until deeply caramelized, about 40 minutes.

② Add the wine and sherry, scraping up any browned bits from the bottom of the pan. Increase the heat to high and cook, stirring constantly, until the liquid evaporates. Reduce the heat to low, stir in the arrowroot starch, and cook for 1 minute.

③ Add the chicken broth, beef broth, thyme, salt, and pepper. Bring to a boil, reduce the heat to medium-low, and simmer for 10 minutes. Remove the thyme.

④ Turn the oven to broil. Fill individual ovenproof bowls with the soup and top each with a toasted bread slice and a slice of cheese. Set the bowls on a baking sheet and broil for 1 to 2 minutes or until the cheese is melted and bubbling.

# HEARTY BEEF STEW

Here's a good old-fashioned stew with rich beef gravy that lets the flavor of the potatoes and carrots come through. This is the perfect hearty dish for a blustery winter day.

① Preheat the oven to 350°F (180°C, or gas mark 4).

② In a zip-top plastic bag, combine the potato starch, sea salt, and black pepper. Add the meat chunks, seal the bag, and toss to coat.

③ In a Dutch oven or other large ovenproof pot over medium-high heat, melt the fat and then brown the meat chunks. Add the onion, celery, and garlic and cook until softened, about 3 to 5 minutes.

④ Stir in the tomato paste, carrots, mushrooms, potatoes, broth, and bay leaf. Bring to a simmer; season with salt and pepper.

⑤ Cover, transfer to the oven, and bake for 3 hours, or until the meat is very tender. Remove the bay leaf before serving.

1 tablespoon (12 g) potato starch

1 teaspoon sea salt, plus more to taste

½ teaspoon ground black pepper, plus more to taste

1 pound (455 g) beef stew meat chunks

2 tablespoons (28 g) cooking fat

1 medium onion, chopped

2 ribs of celery, chopped

2 cloves of garlic, pressed or minced

2 tablespoons (32 g) tomato paste

2 carrots, chopped

8 ounces (225 g) white button mushrooms, halved or quartered

8 ounces (225 g) Yukon gold potatoes, peeled and cut into ½-inch (1.3 cm) cubes (1½ cups [165 g])

4 cups (950 ml) beef broth/ stock (page 93)

1 bay leaf

YIELD: 8 CUPS (1.9 L)

NOTES   Beef stew can be started the day before, refrigerated, and then baked as directed. It can also be cooked in a slow cooker on low for 6 to 8 hours instead of baked.

4 cups (955 ml) chicken broth/stock (page 93)

1 pound (455 g) russet potatoes, peeled and cut into ½-inch (1.3 cm) cubes (3 cups [330 g])

Sea salt, to taste

4 ounces (115 g) nitrate-free bacon, chopped

1 rib of celery, chopped

1 medium onion, chopped

½ of a carrot, peeled and chopped

¼ cup (48 g) potato starch

1 bottle (8 ounces, or 235 ml) clam juice

2 bay leaves

1 sprig of fresh thyme

½ teaspoon white pepper

1 can (6.5 ounces, or 185 g) minced clams, drained and rinsed

1 can (6.5 ounces, or 185 g) chopped clams, drained and rinsed

1 can (12 ounces, or 340 g) whole baby clams, drained and rinsed

2 cups (475 ml) half-and-half (or 1 cup [235 ml] milk and 1 cup [235 ml] heavy cream)

Hot sauce, to taste (such as Tabasco)

YIELD: 8 CUPS (1.9 L)

# CLAM CHOWDER

This clam chowder recipe is easy to make and tastes even better the next day. For an extra hearty chowder, double the clams and garnish with fresh, steamed clams.

---

① In a Dutch oven or large heavy-bottomed pot, bring the broth to a boil. Reduce the heat to medium, add the potatoes and a large pinch of salt, and simmer for about 10 minutes or until the potatoes are tender but not yet completely cooked.

② Drain the potatoes, reserving the cooking liquid. Set both aside.

③ Return the pot to medium heat and cook the bacon pieces until crisp. Add the celery, onion, and carrot. Sauté for 5 minutes or until softened.

④ Add the potato starch, stirring well to coat the vegetables. Add the reserved potato cooking liquid, clam juice, bay leaves, thyme, and pepper. Simmer for 5 minutes or until thick.

⑤ Add the reserved potatoes, clams, and half-and-half. Season with salt, pepper, and a few drops of Tabasco. Return the soup to a simmer (do not boil) for about 3 minutes until heated through. Remove the fresh thyme sprig and bay leaves before serving.

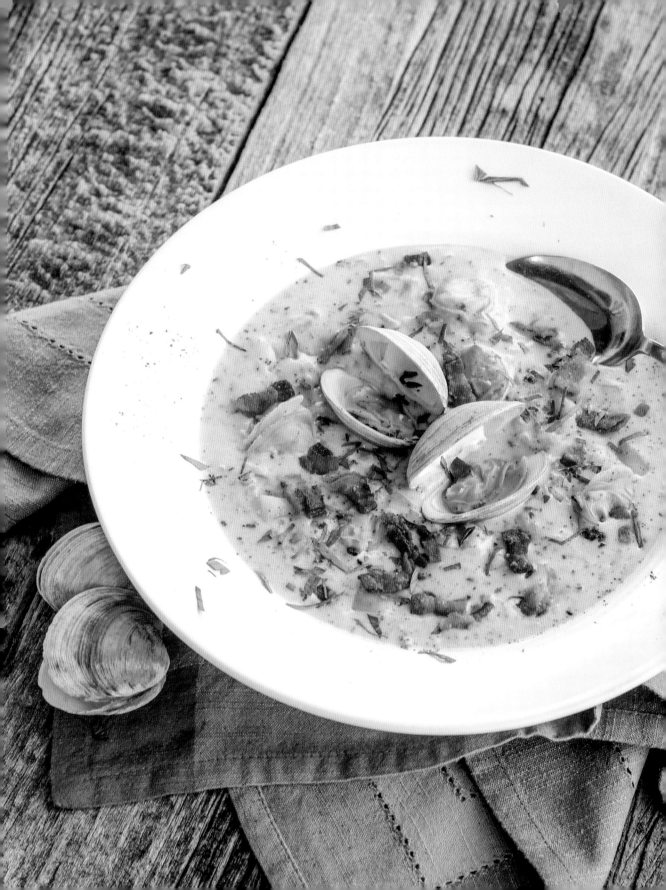

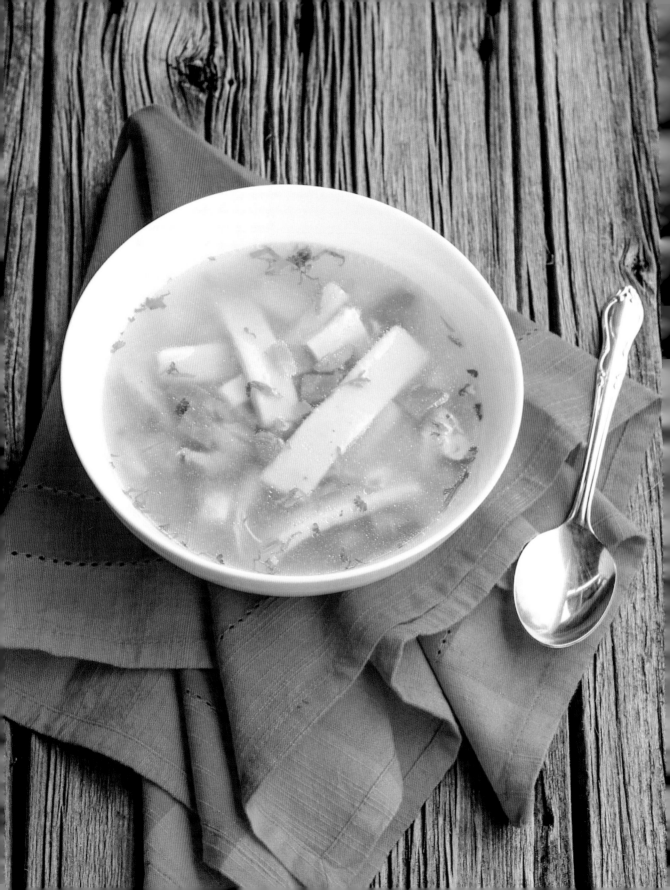

# HOME-STYLE CHICKEN NOODLE SOUP

There is nothing quite like enjoying a bowl of home-style chicken noodle soup. With lots of homemade noodles, it will have everyone asking for seconds.

1 recipe for Pasta Dough (page 37)

Tapioca starch

2 tablespoons (28 g) cooking fat

1 pound (455 g) boneless, skinless chicken breast and/or thighs, cut into bite-size pieces

2 carrots, chopped

1 small onion, chopped

1 rib of celery, sliced

1 clove of garlic, pressed or minced

8 cups (1.9 L) chicken broth/ stock (page 93)

Sea salt and black pepper, to taste

Yield: 10 cups (2.4 L)

① Bring a large pot of salted water to a boil.

② Divide the pasta dough into 4 equal portions. Using additional tapioca starch as needed to avoid sticking, roll out the dough to approximately ¼ inch (6 mm) thick. Use a pizza cutter or knife to cut noodles approximately ½ x 2 inches (1.3 x 5 cm).

③ Boil the noodles for 7 minutes, drain, and rinse with cold water. Set aside.

④ In a large pot over medium heat, melt the fat. Sauté the chicken pieces, carrots, onion, celery, and garlic until the chicken is browned and the vegetables are soft, about 5 minutes. Add the chicken broth and simmer until the chicken is cooked through, about 10 minutes. Reduce the heat to low, add the cooked noodles, and simmer for a few minutes to heat through. Season with salt and pepper.

NOTE Two cups (280 g) of cooked shredded chicken (leftovers or from making bone broth, page 93) can be used in place of the raw chicken pieces. Add the cooked chicken with the noodles instead of with the vegetables and heat through.

2 tablespoons (28 g) cooking fat

1 small onion, finely chopped

1 clove of garlic, pressed or minced

2 tablespoons (24 g) potato starch

2 cups (475 ml) chicken broth/stock (page 93)

3 tablespoons (48 g) tomato paste

2 tablespoons (28 ml) Worcestershire sauce

¼ teaspoon seafood seasoning (such as Old Bay)

Pinch of cayenne pepper

2 cups (475 ml) heavy cream

1 pound (455 g) lump crabmeat, canned or fresh

Sea salt and white pepper, to taste

YIELD: 8 CUPS (1.9 L)

# CRAB BISQUE

It's almost surprising that such a rich and delicious crab bisque can be made in less than 30 minutes, and it isn't thickened with grains! It can also be made with a combination of crab, shrimp, and lobster to make a seafood bisque, if desired.

① In a large pot over medium heat, melt the fat. Sauté the onion and garlic until soft, about 2 to 4 minutes. Sprinkle the potato starch over the vegetables and whisk in the broth until combined with no lumps.

② Add the tomato paste, Worcestershire sauce, seafood seasoning, and cayenne pepper and stir to combine. Reduce the heat to low and add the cream. Gently add in the crabmeat, being careful not to completely break up the chunks of meat. Simmer for 5 minutes or until heated through. Season with the salt and pepper.

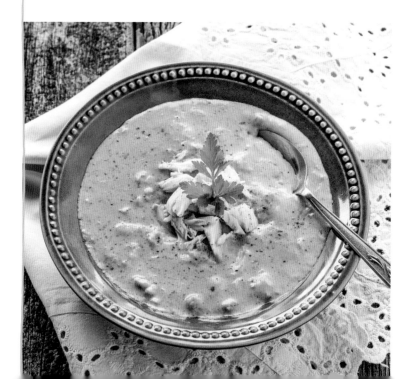

# ITALIAN WEDDING SOUP

Luckily you don't have to be Italian to love this easy-to-make soup! Homemade mini meatballs simmered in homemade broth with strings of cooked egg and fresh cooked greens results in a comforting soup that really hits the spot.

2 tablespoons (28 g) cooking fat

2 carrots, chopped

1 small onion, chopped

1 rib of celery, sliced

1 clove of garlic, pressed or minced

8 cups (1.9 L) chicken broth/stock (page 93)

½ of a recipe for uncooked meatball mixture (page 135)

4 cups coarsely chopped (200 g) fresh escarole, (120 g) spinach, or (268 g) kale

2 large eggs

⅓ cup (33 g) grated Parmesan or Romano cheese

YIELD: 10 CUPS (2.4 L)

① In a large pot over medium heat, melt the fat. Sauté the carrots, onion, celery, and garlic until softened, about 5 minutes. Add the chicken broth and bring to a simmer.

② Meanwhile, roll teaspoon-size portions of the meatball mixture into balls and drop into the soup. Reduce the heat to low, cover, and cook for 20 minutes or until the meatballs are cooked through.

③ Once the meatballs are cooked through, add the chopped greens and cook for an additional 2 minutes or until wilted.

④ Just before serving, bring the soup to a gentle simmer. In a small bowl, beat together the eggs and Parmesan cheese. While stirring the soup constantly, slowly pour in the egg mixture. The residual heat will cook the ribbons of egg throughout the soup.

# Chapter 7:

# MAIN MEALS

MAIN DISHES make up the largest part of a food budget and they are, potentially, where the most adjustment is needed when going grain-free, both in what to cook and in how to cook it. My best tip to ease the transition and stay the course is to create a weekly meal plan with a shopping list that utilizes what you already have on hand that needs to be eaten, considers what is the best value (seasonal, fresh, on sale, etc.), and taps in to what you are craving. For example, using up ground beef and cabbage you already have in Cabbage Rolls in Tomato Sauce (page 119) on Monday and satisfying your craving for New York–Style Pizza (page 152) on Tuesday is a surefire way to help keep you on track.

But aside from a mere shopping list, a meal plan can be a valuable tool for remaining grain-free. Here's why:

**It saves money.** Creating a meal plan helps you stick to a budget. When you plan out your meals and make a weekly shopping list, you are more likely to buy only what is needed, and you will make fewer trips to the grocery store. You can also make the most of fresh, seasonal produce, which always costs less.

I most often plan one meal one night and use part of it for several other meals over the next few days. Most Mondays I roast a whole chicken in my slow cooker and then serve it with green beans and mashed potatoes and gravy (page 120). I pick the meat off the bones to use for

chicken salads, Creamed Chicken and Biscuits (page 123), Southwest Quesadillas (page 78), or Fajitas (page 141) for lunches and dinners. Then I put the bones back into the slow cooker to make bone broth (page 93). One chicken will feed us for several meals *plus* make a few quarts (L) of nutrient-dense broth.

**It reduces stress.** There is nothing worse than leaving work and stressing on the drive home about what you are going to cook for dinner. Having a meal plan means that you know exactly what you need to do when you get home, taking the stress out of getting dinner on the table. Knowing that everything you need to make a 30-minute dinner is waiting at home in the fridge will set your mind at ease!

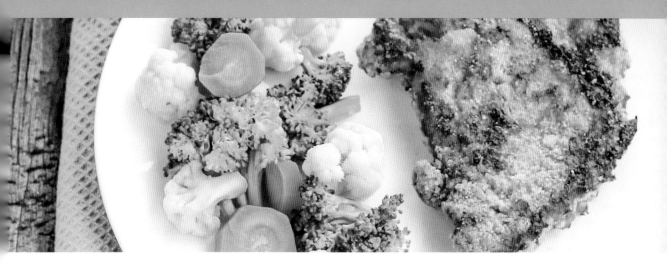

**It saves time.** Spending just half an hour each week planning meals and organizing my shopping list saves the time I would spend each day wondering what to cook for dinner. It might not be this quick when you first plan your meals, but once you get into a routine, it will take you no time at all.

Meal planning also allows you to cook in bulk to make extra for another day. I find it's not much more work to double or triple a recipe because I've already got my ingredients out and made a mess in the kitchen. In the summer when our garden is overflowing with tomatoes and green peppers, I'll make several batches of Stuffed Peppers (page 112) and package them in meal-size containers for the freezer.

**It creates healthier meals.** When you have a meal plan, you can plan to serve your family healthy meals that are nutritious, rather than just throwing something together at the last minute without taking into account the nutrients that your family is getting from the meal. You can prep on the weekends or the night before to make it easier.

Most often, when people "cheat" on their grain-free diet, it's when they are not prepared and are craving foods from their past. Having grain-free recipes for your favorite foods as part of your regular diet will prevent you from sabotaging your health with a trip to the drive-through.

**It produces less waste.** According to the Environmental Protection Agency, food leftovers are the single largest component of the waste stream by weight in the United States. Many people cook enough food that there are frequently leftovers, but the food often just sits in the fridge and goes bad instead of being eaten. Planning your meals makes it easy to create meals that either make just enough or provide leftovers for lunch or even freezer meals. For example, making Turkey Pot Pies (page 114) with your leftover Thanksgiving turkey and putting them in the freezer for later is a great way to use up leftovers that most people get tired of eating and tend to waste. Come February, you'll be excited to have those pies and leftover turkey to eat!

# STUFFED PEPPERS

4 to 8 green or colored bell peppers (4 extra-large or 8 small peppers)

2 tablespoons (28 g) cooking fat

1 small onion, chopped

1 clove of garlic, minced or pressed

½ of a carrot, grated

2 tablespoons (32 g) tomato paste

1 cup (100 g) raw Cauliflower Rice (page 35)

1 pound (455 g) ground beef

1 teaspoon dried parsley or 1 tablespoon (4 g) fresh, chopped

1 teaspoon sea salt

½ teaspoon ground black pepper

½ cup (50 g) grated Parmesan cheese, divided

4 cups (980 g) tomato sauce or tomato soup

YIELD: 4 SERVINGS

When I went to college, the first meal I remember making was my mom's stuffed peppers. All my sisters in the sorority house were drawn to the kitchen by the delicious smell. I make them the same way today, only using Cauliflower Rice (page 35) in place of white rice. Because these are made with a pound (455 g) of ground beef, they will serve four adults each with a 4-ounce (115 g) serving. The recipe can made using four extra-large peppers (one per serving) or eight small peppers (two per serving), based on what size peppers you have available.

## MAKE IT A MEAL

Serve the peppers with tossed salad and mashed potatoes or sweet potatoes.

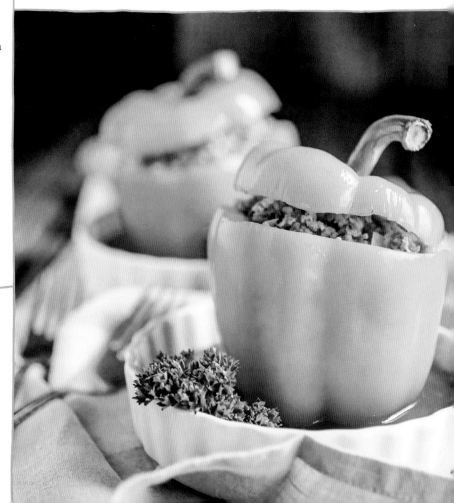

① Preheat the oven to 350°F (180°C, or gas mark 4).

② Slice off the tops of the peppers about ½ inch (1.3 cm) down from the stems, reserving the tops for another use, if desired. Remove and discard the seeds and cores. If any of the peppers won't stand upright, slice a little off the bottom, making sure not to cut into the cavity. Arrange the peppers in a Dutch oven or an ovenproof casserole dish.

③ Melt the cooking fat in a medium skillet over medium heat. Add the onion and garlic. Cook, stirring occasionally, until they begin to soften, about 5 minutes. Add the carrot, tomato paste, and cauliflower rice, tossing to coat. Cook for 1 minute. Remove the vegetable mixture from the heat and allow to cool slightly.

④ In a large bowl, combine the beef with the parsley, salt, pepper, ¼ cup (25 g) of the Parmesan cheese, and the vegetable mixture. Divide the mixture among the bell pepper shells and then pour the tomato sauce over the stuffed peppers.

⑤ Cover with foil and bake until the peppers are tender and the filling is hot, about 1 hour. Sprinkle with the remaining ¼ cup (25 g) cheese and bake until the cheese is melted, about 1 minute more. Remove from the oven and let the peppers rest for 5 minutes prior to serving.

NOTES   Raw stuffed peppers can be prepared up to 2 days ahead and stored in the refrigerator. Raw or cooked, they can also be frozen for up to 6 months. In the summer months when peppers are plentiful, make up several batches, package in meal-size portions, and freeze. Thaw frozen stuffed peppers in the refrigerator overnight prior to baking.

¼ cup (55 g) cooking fat

1 small onion, chopped

1 rib of celery, chopped

1 clove of garlic, pressed
   or minced

2 tablespoons (24 g) potato
   starch

4 cups (950 ml) chicken
   broth/stock (page 93)

2 cups (approximately
   240 g total) fresh or frozen
   vegetables (carrots, green
   beans, peas, lima beans,
   etc.), diced if necessary

2 cups (280 g) shredded
   cooked turkey or chicken

¼ cup (60 ml) heavy cream

Sea salt and black pepper,
   to taste

1 recipe for Pie Crust
   (page 33)

YIELD: ONE 9-INCH (23 CM) POT PIE
OR FOUR 6-INCH (15 CM)
INDIVIDUAL POT PIES

NOTES   This recipe can be
made into 4 individual (6-inch,
or 15 cm) pot pies. Assembled
and unbaked pot pies can be
covered with plastic wrap and
frozen. Bake frozen pot pies,
minus the plastic, for 1 hour at
400°F (200°C, or gas mark 6) or
until cooked through and the
filling is bubbly.

# TURKEY POT PIE

When we first got married, my husband loved those
individual frozen pot pies. I learned to make them from
scratch and made them for years. I still make them
regularly, only now without grain.

①  Preheat the oven to 350°F (180°C, or gas mark 4).

②  In a 2-quart (2 L) saucepan over medium heat, melt the fat.
Sauté the onion, celery, and garlic for about 5 minutes or until
soft. Sprinkle the potato starch over the veggies and mix well.
Slowly pour in the chicken stock, whisking until smooth, with
no starch clumps.

③  Add the vegetables. Raise the heat and bring to a boil. Reduce
the heat to medium-low and simmer until the veggies are cooked
and the broth has thickened, about 3 to 4 minutes. Add the turkey
and cream and season with the salt and pepper. Remove from the
heat and allow to cool slightly.

④  Roll out the pie dough and lay the bottom crust in a 9-inch
(23 cm) pie plate.

⑤  Pour the filling into the pie crust. Roll out the top crust and then
cover the pie. Press, using your fingers or the tines of a fork, to seal
the edges, and cut away any excess dough. Make several small slits
in the top to allow steam to escape.

⑥  Place the pie on a baking sheet (to catch any drips) and bake for
35 to 45 minutes or until the pastry is golden brown and the filling
is bubbly. Cool for 10 minutes before serving.

# SLOPPY JOE BAKED POTATOES

A sloppy Joe sandwich is an American classic made of ground beef in a seasoned tomato sauce served on a hamburger bun, originating in the early 1900s. For a healthier version, I've eliminated the bun and made our sloppy Joe sauce from scratch (which eliminates any grain-containing thickeners commonly found in processed sauces) and served it on a baked potato for a delicious twist the whole family will enjoy. Of course, you can make a sloppy Joe sandwich using my Sliceable Sandwich Bread (page 38), if you prefer.

1 pound (455 g) ground beef

1 small onion, chopped

½ of a green bell pepper, chopped

2 cloves of garlic, pressed or minced

½ cup (120 g) ketchup

1 tablespoon (20 g) honey

2 teaspoons chili powder

1 teaspoon dry mustard powder

1 teaspoon Worcestershire sauce

Pinch of crushed red pepper flakes

Sea salt and black pepper, to taste

4 russet potatoes, baked

## YIELD: 4 SERVINGS

① In a large skillet over medium heat, cook the beef, onion, green pepper, and garlic for 3 to 4 minutes, until soft. Reduce the heat to low and add the ketchup, honey, chili powder, mustard, Worcestershire sauce, and red pepper.

② Simmer for about 5 minutes for the flavors to combine, seasoning with salt and pepper. Split open the baked potatoes. Divide the Sloppy Joe mixture evenly among the potatoes, scooping it on top of each.

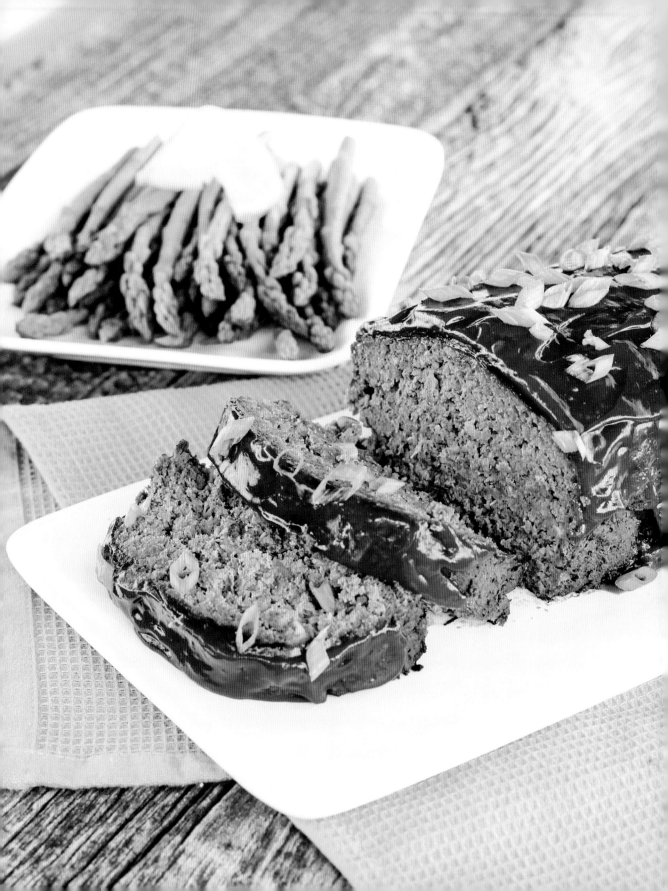

# CLASSIC MEATLOAF

Everyone needs a classic meatloaf recipe in his or her meal rotation. This moist and delicious version uses mushrooms in place of bread to give it a soft texture. But don't worry if mushrooms aren't your favorite: I've tricked many mushroom haters with this meatloaf.

½ cup (120 g) ketchup

½ cup (96 g) coconut sugar

½ cup (120 ml) apple cider vinegar

1 large carrot, peeled and grated

1 large onion, chopped

2 cloves of garlic, pressed or minced

1 pound (455 g) white button mushrooms

¼ cup (16 g) chopped fresh parsley

2 tablespoons (28 g) cooking fat

1 teaspoon sea salt

½ teaspoon ground black pepper

1½ pounds (680 g) ground pork

1 pound (455 g) ground beef

¼ cup (28 g) blanched almond flour

## YIELD: 8 TO 10 SERVINGS

① Preheat the oven to 350°F (180°C, or gas mark 4).

② In a small saucepan over medium heat, combine the ketchup, sugar, and vinegar. Simmer for 10 minutes, stirring occasionally.

③ Meanwhile, in a food processor, combine the carrot, onion, garlic, mushrooms, and parsley and pulse to chop finely.

④ In a large skillet over medium heat, melt the fat. Sauté the vegetable mixture until cooked through, about 3 to 4 minutes. Season with the salt and pepper, add 3 tablespoons (45 g) of the ketchup mixture, and allow to cool.

⑤ In a large-size bowl, combine the pork, beef, cooled veggie mixture, and almond flour. Mix well. Press the meatloaf mixture into a 4½ x 8½-inch (11.4 x 21.6 cm) loaf pan, and spread the remaining ketchup mixture on top.

⑥ Bake for 90 minutes. Allow the cooked meatloaf to rest for at least 30 minutes prior to removing from the pan and slicing.

## MAKE IT A MEAL
Serve with mashed potatoes and steamed asparagus.

# CABBAGE ROLLS IN TOMATO SAUCE

Stuffed cabbage, also known as haluski or halupki, was a family favorite for both my husband and me. Our grandmothers made them regularly, and I've come up with my own version that is a perfect combination of our two families' recipes, made without grain.

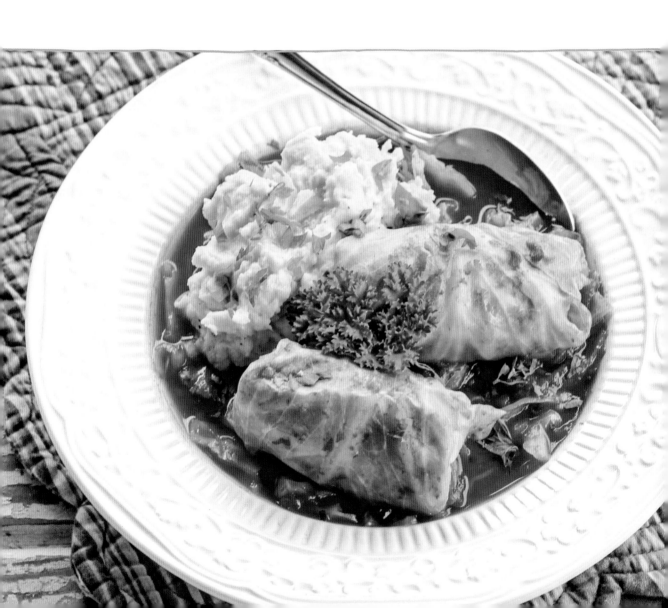

1. Preheat the oven to 350°F (180°C, or gas mark 4).

2. Fill a large pot about halfway with water and bring to a boil. Submerge the whole head of cabbage into the water and boil until it is al dente and the outer leaves can be peeled off without breaking, about 10 to 15 minutes. Set aside to cool.

3. In a large bowl, combine the beef, cauliflower rice, parsley, onion powder, salt, garlic powder, and pepper. Use your hands to mix well.

4. Gently peel the outer 8 leaves off the head of cabbage and reserve for the cabbage rolls. With a sharp knife, shave off any thick veins from the outside of the reserved cabbage leaves. Quarter the head of cabbage, cut out the core from each quarter, and place in a Dutch oven or 2-quart (2 L) casserole dish.

5. Lay a cabbage leaf out in front of you so that where it was connected at the core is toward you and curling up. Place one-eighth of the meat mixture about 2 inches (5 cm) from the edge closest to you and shape the meat into a 3-inch (7.5 cm)-wide log. Fold the 2 inches (5 cm) closest to you over the top of the meat and roll it so that the edge is underneath the meat. Next, fold the left and right sides of the leaf over the meat (you can trim the sides if there are more than 2 to 3 inches [5 to 7.5 cm] of cabbage). Roll the meat forward, toward the farthest edge.

6. Place the cabbage rolls, seam-side down, in the Dutch oven with the cabbage quarters. Pour the tomatoes and juice over the top and sprinkle with additional salt and pepper. Cover and bake for 2 hours or until the rolls are so tender you don't need a knife to cut them.

**1 medium head of cabbage**

**1 pound (455 g) ground beef**

**1½ cups (150 g) raw Cauliflower Rice (page 35)**

**⅓ cup (21 g) chopped fresh parsley**

**1 teaspoon onion powder**

**1 teaspoon sea salt**

**½ teaspoon garlic powder**

**¼ teaspoon ground black pepper**

**4 cups (720 g) canned chopped or diced tomatoes in juice**

## YIELD: 4 SERVINGS

## MAKE IT A MEAL
Serve with mashed potatoes.

## FOR STEAK:

2 tablespoons (28 g) cooking fat

8 ounces (225 g) white button mushrooms, chopped

1 medium onion, chopped

2 cloves of garlic, pressed or minced

1 teaspoon sea salt

½ teaspoon ground black pepper

1 pound (455 g) ground beef

1 large egg

1 tablespoon (7 g) coconut flour

1 teaspoon dried parsley or 1 tablespoon (4 g) chopped fresh parsley

## FOR GRAVY:

2 tablespoons (28 g) cooking fat

8 ounces (225 g) white button mushrooms, sliced

Juice of 1 lemon wedge

½ teaspoon garlic powder

Pinch of sea salt

¼ cup (48 g) potato starch

3 cups (700 ml) beef broth/ stock (page 93)

YIELD: 4 SERVINGS

# SALISBURY STEAK WITH MUSHROOM GRAVY

Growing up, my mom's Salisbury steak with mushroom gravy was my favorite meal. She always served it with buttered broccoli and mashed potatoes.

① To make the steak: In a large, straight-sided skillet with a lid, over medium heat, melt the fat. Sauté the mushrooms, onion, garlic, sea salt, and pepper until the mushrooms have released their liquid and it has evaporated (to a nearly dry skillet), about 5 to 7 minutes. Transfer to a food processor and puree.

② In a large bowl, combine the pureed vegetable mixture with the beef, egg, flour, and parsley, using your hands to mix well. Divide into 8 equal portions and form into patties about 1 inch (2.5 cm) thick. Return them to the same skillet the vegetables were cooked in and cook over medium heat for about 15 minutes or until cooked through. (If your ground beef is very lean, you may need to add a little additional fat to prevent sticking.) Removed the cooked patties from the skillet and set aside.

③ To make the gravy: Return the skillet to medium heat and add the fat. Sauté the mushrooms, lemon juice, garlic powder, and salt until the mushrooms and vegetables are cooked and soft, about 5 minutes. Add the starch and mix well to coat. Add the beef broth and whisk until smooth, with no clumps of starch.

④ Put the patties into the gravy and cover the skillet with a lid. Simmer over low heat for about 10 minutes or until the gravy is thickened and the patties are heated through.

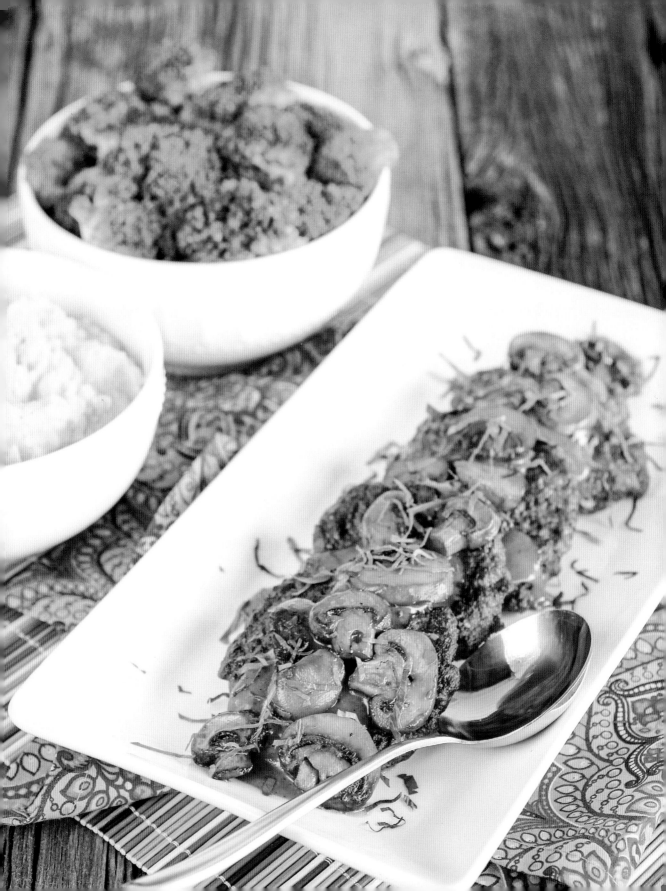

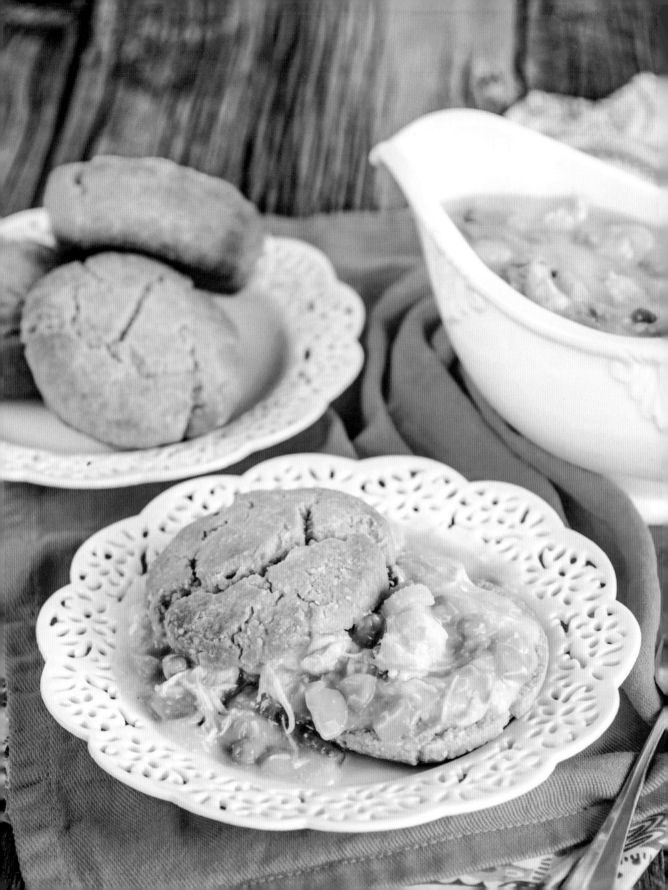

# CREAMED CHICKEN AND BISCUITS

This homemade chicken and biscuits dish will satisfy any craving for comfort food. The chicken stew is rich and creamy, and the grain-free biscuits serve as the perfect complement.

① In a 2-quart (2 L) saucepan over medium heat, melt the fat. Sauté the onion, celery, and garlic for about 5 minutes until soft. Sprinkle the potato starch over the veggies and mix well. Slowly pour in the stock, whisking until smooth, with no clumps of starch.

② Add the vegetables. Raise the heat and bring to a boil. Lower the heat to medium-low and simmer until the veggies are soft and the broth has thickened, about 5 minutes. Add the chicken and heavy cream and season with salt and pepper. Cook, stirring gently, until heated through, about 3 minutes.

③ Serve each person 1 halved biscuit topped with the chicken gravy.

¼ cup (55 g) cooking fat

1 small onion, chopped

1 rib of celery, chopped

1 clove of garlic, pressed or minced

2 tablespoons (24 g) potato starch

4 cups (950 ml) chicken broth/stock (page 93)

2 cups (approximately 240 g total) fresh or frozen vegetables (carrots, green beans, peas, lima beans, etc.), diced if necessary

2 cups (280 g) shredded or chopped cooked chicken

¼ cup (60 ml) heavy cream

Sea salt and black pepper, to taste

4 Buttermilk Biscuits (page 43), halved

## YIELD: 4 SERVINGS

## MAKE IT A MEAL
Serve with a tossed salad.

# EGGPLANT PARMESAN STACKS

This is a unique spin on a classic Italian baked eggplant Parmesan, made into individual stacks of grain-free breaded eggplant slices layered with cheese and tomato sauce. Zucchini may be used in place of eggplant, if you're not a fan of eggplant or they are unavailable (prepare the same way). Zucchini Parmesan stacks are just as good—if not better.

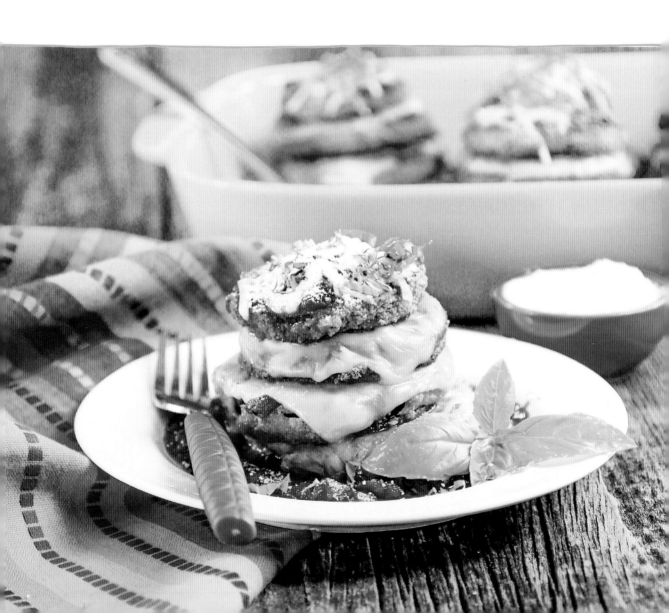

① Preheat the oven to 350°F (180°C, or gas mark 4). Place several layers of paper towels on a baking sheet.

② Slice the eggplants crosswise into ⅓-inch (8 mm)-thick slices and arrange in a single layer on the paper towels. Sprinkle lightly with the salt and allow to rest for 30 minutes to release any water.

③ Using 3 shallow bowls, fill one with the tapioca starch, one with the beaten eggs, and one with a mixture of the Parmesan cheese, breading mix, and Italian seasoning.

④ In a Dutch oven or other large heavy-bottomed pot, heat 2 to 3 inches (5 to 7.5 cm) of fat to 350°F (180°C).

⑤ Bread the eggplant slices by dredging in the tapioca, then the egg, then the breading mixture. Make sure each slice is completely coated.

⑥ Fry the eggplant slices in batches for 1 to 2 minutes per side or until brown and crispy. Drain on a paper towel–lined plate.

⑦ Spread 1 cup (245 g) of the marinara sauce in the bottom of a 9 x 13-inch (23 x 33 cm) casserole dish. Create 6 to 8 stacks of eggplant Parmesan, alternating a slice of eggplant, a spoonful of sauce, and a sprinkle of mozzarella and provolone for 3 or 4 layers in each stack. Pour any remaining sauce around the stacks.

⑧ Bake for 30 minutes or until heated through and the cheese is melted.

**2 medium eggplants**

**Sea salt**

**1 cup (120 g) tapioca starch**

**3 large eggs**

**1 cup (100 g) grated Parmesan cheese**

**1 cup (115 g) Breading Mix (page 34)**

**1 teaspoon Italian seasoning**

**Lard or palm oil, for frying**

**4 cups (980 g) tomato/ marinara sauce**

**2 cups (230 g) shredded mozzarella cheese**

**2 cups (230 g) shredded provolone cheese**

## YIELD: 4 TO 6 SERVINGS

## MAKE IT A MEAL

Serve with a tossed salad, grilled chicken, and spaghetti squash.

- 2 tablespoons (21 g) arrowroot starch
- ½ teaspoon sea salt
- ½ teaspoon garlic powder
- ½ teaspoon onion powder
- ¼ teaspoon ground black pepper
- 1 pound (455 g) sirloin steak, cut into ½ x 2-inch (1.3 x 5 cm) strips
- 2 tablespoons (28 g) cooking fat
- 8 ounces (225 g) white button mushrooms, sliced
- 1 medium onion, sliced
- 2 cloves of garlic, pressed or minced
- 2 cups (475 ml) beef broth/stock (page 93)
- ¼ cup (60 ml) heavy cream
- 2 medium zucchini
- Optional garnish: sour cream and chopped fresh parsley

## YIELD: 4 SERVINGS

# BEEF STROGANOFF WITH "ZOODLES"

This family favorite is your classic beef stroganoff, only served with thinly sliced zucchini instead of noodles.

① In a large bowl, combine the starch, salt, powders, and pepper. Add the beef strips and toss to coat.

② In a large skillet over medium heat, melt the fat. Brown the meat strips, about 5 minutes. Add the mushrooms, onion, and garlic, and sauté for 2 to 3 minutes until the vegetables are soft.

③ Stir in the broth and bring to a boil. Reduce the heat to low, cover, and simmer for 20 minutes. Remove from the heat, stir in the heavy cream, and season with additional sea salt and pepper, to taste. Replace the lid and allow to rest.

④ Wash and remove the ends of the zucchinis. Cut into thin zucchini noodles (aka "zoodles") using a spiralizer, julienne peeler, or mandoline. Add 1 to 2 cups (235 to 475 ml) of water to a pot fitted with a steamer insert. Bring the water to a boil over high heat, place the zoodles in the steamer basket, cover with the lid, and steam for 1 minute.

⑤ Serve the beef stroganoff on top of the zoodles, garnished with a dollop of sour cream and fresh parsley, if desired.

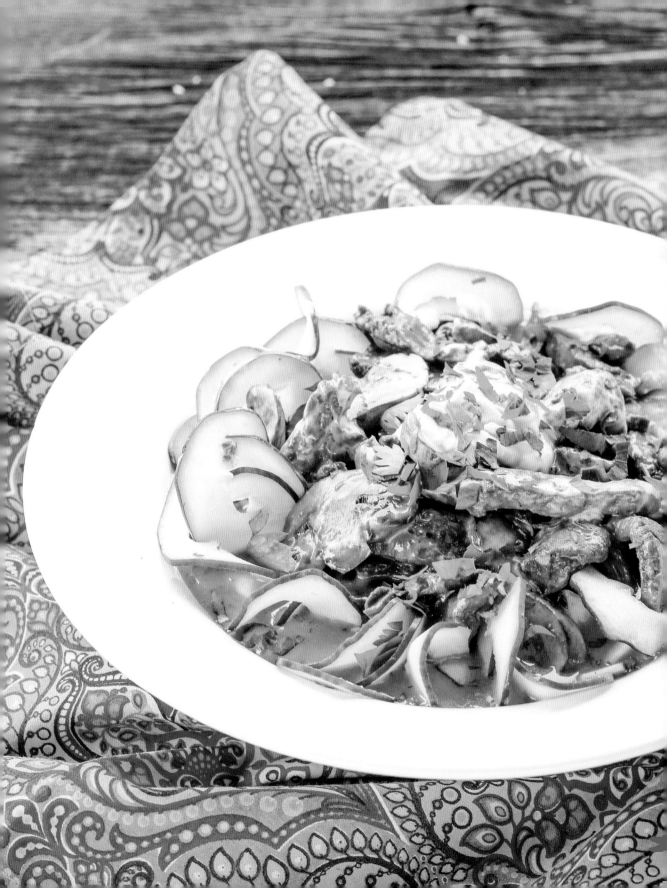

½ cup (56 g) blanched almond flour

½ cup (64 g) arrowroot starch

1 teaspoon onion powder

1 teaspoon garlic powder

1 teaspoon dried parsley

½ teaspoon sea salt

¼ teaspoon ground black pepper

Optional: ¼ teaspoon cayenne pepper

4 bone-in pork chops (4 to 6 ounces, or 115 to 170 g each)

## YIELD: 4 SERVINGS

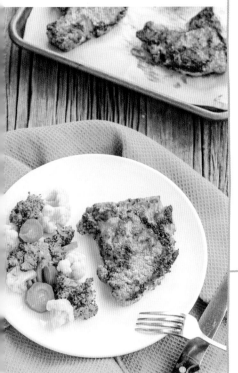

# CRISPY BAKED PORK CHOPS

Just as easy as can be: shake your pork chops in a breading mix and bake until crispy. Feel free to use chicken in place of the pork for an equally delicious dish.

① Preheat the oven to 400°F (200°C, or gas mark 6) and line a baking sheet with parchment paper.

② In a 1-gallon (3.8 L) zip-top plastic bag, add the flour, starch, powders, parsley, salt, black pepper, and cayenne pepper, if using. Shake well to combine.

③ Lightly moisten the pork chops with water and then place in the bag of breading mix, seal, and shake to coat. Set the chops on the prepared baking sheet.

④ Bake the breaded pork chops for 30 minutes or until cooked through and crispy.

## MAKE IT A MEAL
Serve with baked sweet potatoes and steamed Brussels sprouts.

# CHICKEN-FRIED STEAK WITH COUNTRY GRAVY

Chicken-fried steak has a few other names throughout the world, such as country-fried steak, pan-fried steak, Wiener schnitzel, and milanese. It is tenderized ("cubed") top round, made like fried chicken, and served with a milk gravy made from the drippings left in the pan. The steak, when fried, should look just like the coating on a piece of Southern fried chicken.

**4 cube steaks or tenderized round steaks (4 ounces, or 115 g each)**

**1 teaspoon sea salt, divided**

**½ teaspoon ground black pepper, divided**

**1½ cups (173 g) Breading Mix (page 34)**

**2 large eggs**

**¼ cup (55 g) cooking fat**

**1 cup (235 ml) milk**

## Yield: 4 servings

① Season the meat with ½ teaspoon of the salt and ¼ teaspoon of the pepper; set aside.

② In a shallow dish, combine the breading mix with the remaining ½ teaspoon salt and ¼ teaspoon pepper; reserve 2 tablespoons (14 g) of the mixture. In a separate shallow dish, lightly beat the eggs. Dredge each steak in the dry mixture. Dip in the beaten egg and then dredge in the dry mixture again.

③ Arrange the breaded steaks on 2 wax paper–lined plate(s) and freeze for a minimum of 30 minutes.

④ Heat the fat in a large skillet over medium-high heat. Fry the steaks for 3 to 4 minutes on each side or until golden brown and cooked through. Drain on paper towels.

⑤ Pour off all but 2 tablespoons (28 g) of the fat. Sprinkle the reserved 2 tablespoons (14 g) dredging mixture onto the fat. Cook over medium heat for 1 minute, stirring constantly. Gradually whisk in the milk, scraping up any browned bits from the bottom of the skillet. Cook, stirring frequently, for 3 to 4 minutes or until the gravy is thickened and bubbly. Season with additional salt and pepper, to taste. Serve the steaks with the gravy.

## MAKE IT A MEAL

Serve with mashed potatoes and steamed green beans.

1 large egg

⅓ cup (80 ml) water

1 tablespoon (14 g) cooking fat, melted

1 cup (115 g) Breading Mix (page 34)

Lard or palm oil, for frying

2 large-size potatoes, thinly sliced

4 wild-caught white fish fillets (4 ounces, or 115 g each) or 1 pound (454 g), cut into 4 even pieces (Perch, flounder, or cod are good choices.)

Sea salt, to taste

YIELD: 4 SERVINGS

# BATTERED FISH AND CHIPS

Grilled, broiled, and baked are all good choices when it comes to preparing fish. However, none of these preparations beats a good batter-dipped fried fish.

① In a large shallow dish or a pie plate, whisk together the egg, water, and fat. Add the breading mix and whisk well to remove any lumps.

② In a Dutch oven or other large heavy-bottomed pot, heat 2 to 3 inches (5 to 7.5 cm) of fat to 350°F (180°C).

③ Working in batches, if necessary, fry thin slices of potatoes until they stop sizzling, about 3 to 5 minutes. Using a slotted spoon, remove the potatoes from the fat and drain on a paper towel–lined plate.

④ Dip each piece of fish into the batter, allowing the excess to drain off. Fry the battered fish, turning once, until cooked through and golden brown, about 3 minutes per side, depending on the thickness. Drain on a paper towel–lined plate and season with the salt.

⑤ Quickly return the potatoes to the fat for 30 seconds to make them extra crispy. Remove from the fat, drain on a paper towel–lined plate, and season with the salt. Serve the fish and chips with Homemade Tartar Sauce (page 143).

## MAKE IT A MEAL

Serve with coleslaw and pickles.

# BUTTERMILK FRIED CHICKEN

The addition of buttermilk to the grain-free breading gives this recipe a twist to make it different from other fried chicken recipes. For extra tender and flavorful chicken, marinate it in another 2 cups (475 ml) buttermilk overnight in the refrigerator before breading.

2 cups (230 g) Breading Mix (page 34)

1 teaspoon paprika

¼ teaspoon cayenne pepper

2 cups (475 ml) cultured buttermilk

1 cut-up fryer chicken, skin on

Lard or palm oil, for frying

YIELD: 4 SERVINGS

① In a large bowl, combine the breading mix, paprika, and cayenne pepper. Pour the buttermilk into a shallow dish or pie plate.

② Bread each piece of chicken by dredging it in the breading mix and then dipping it in the buttermilk and back into the dry mix to coat heavily with breading (dry, wet, dry). Place the breaded chicken pieces on a wax paper–lined plate(s) and place in the freezer for 30 minutes.

③ Preheat the oven to 350°F (180°C, or gas mark 4).

④ Heat 1½ inches (3.8 cm) of fat in a deep skillet or Dutch oven over medium-high heat to 350°F (180°C).

⑤ Add the chicken to the oil, 2 or 3 pieces at a time. Do not crowd the pan. Cover the pan and fry for about 5 minutes, checking to make sure the chicken isn't getting too brown. Turn the chicken over to cook the other side, cover, and fry for an additional 5 minutes. (The chicken will continue to cook in the oven.)

⑥ Carefully place the fried pieces of chicken on a baking sheet and bake for 10 to 15 minutes until the chicken is cooked through to an internal temperature of at least 160°F (71°C).

NOTES  One cut-up fryer chicken is equal to 2 wings, 2 bone-in breasts, 2 thighs, and 2 legs. Feel free to use any equivalent cuts as desired.

1 cup (250 g) ricotta cheese

2 large eggs

½ cup (50 g) grated
   Parmesan cheese

1 teaspoon sea salt

1 teaspoon white pepper

1 teaspoon garlic powder

½ cup (56 g) blanched
   almond flour

½ cup (64 g) arrowroot starch

½ cup (60 g) tapioca starch,
   divided

**FOR SAUTÉ:**

2 tablespoons (28 g) butter
   or ghee

1 clove of garlic, pressed
   or minced

8 cups (240 g) fresh spinach

1 pint (300 g) cherry
   tomatoes, halved

½ cup (75 g) crumbled
   feta cheese

## YIELD: 4 SERVINGS

## MAKE IT A MEAL

Serve with a tossed salad and
grilled chicken.

# RICOTTA GNOCCHI WITH SPINACH, TOMATOES, AND FETA

A traditional Florentine pasta, ricotta gnocchi is the
lighter version of northern Italy's potato gnocchi—made
even healthier by substituting almond flour for the
traditional all-purpose flour. This gnocchi cooks up as
soft, mild-flavored dumplings. They are delicious with
any type of sauce you'd usually serve on pasta.

① To make the gnocchi: In a large bowl, stir together the ricotta,
eggs, Parmesan cheese, salt, pepper, and garlic powder until
evenly combined.

② Mix in the almond flour, arrowroot starch, and ¼ cup (30 g) of
the tapioca starch to form a soft dough. Add more of the remaining
¼ cup (30 g) tapioca starch as needed.

③ Line a baking sheet with waxed paper and lightly dust the
paper with tapioca starch. Divide the dough into 4 equal pieces. On
a surface dusted with tapioca starch, roll each piece into a ½-inch
(1.3 cm)-thick rope. Cut each rope into 1-inch (2.5 cm) pieces and
place on the prepared baking sheet. Place the gnocchi in the
refrigerator until ready to cook.

④ Bring a large pot of lightly salted water to a boil over high heat.
Boil the gnocchi, in batches if necessary, until they float to the
surface, 1 to 2 minutes. Drain or remove from the water with
a skimmer.

⑤ To make the sauté: In a large skillet over medium heat, melt the
butter. Sauté the garlic until fragrant, about 1 minute. Add the
gnocchi, spinach, and tomatoes. Cook, stirring, for 2 to 3 minutes or
until heated through and combined. Sprinkle with the feta cheese
just before serving.

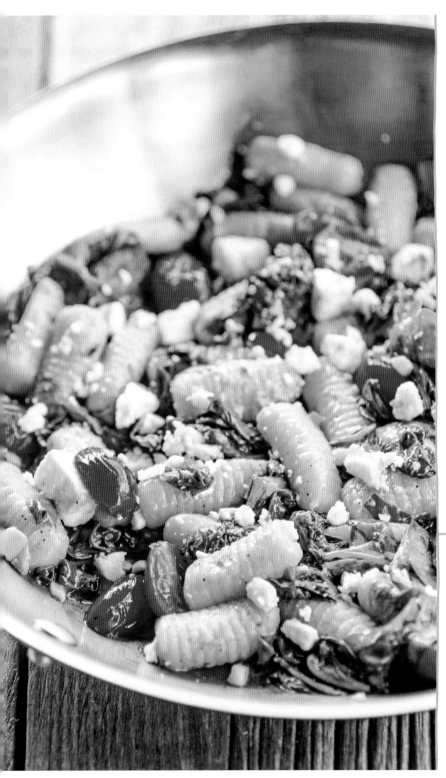

**NOTE** Gnocchi can be made ahead and frozen, uncooked. Freeze them individually on a wax paper–lined baking sheet and then transfer them to a plastic bag or sealed container once frozen. Cook frozen gnocchi the same as fresh; the cooking time may be extended a couple of minutes.

## FOR AIOLI:

½ cup (115 g) mayonnaise

Juice of 1 lemon wedge

1 teaspoon ground
  horseradish

1 teaspoon chopped fresh dill

⅛ teaspoon ground black
  pepper

Sea salt, to taste

## FOR PATTIES:

12 ounces (340 g) canned
  boneless, skinless salmon

4 scallions, chopped

¼ of a red bell pepper, finely
  chopped

¼ cup (60 g) mayonnaise

Juice of 2 lemon wedges

2 tablespoons (14 g) coconut
  flour

1 clove of garlic, minced
  or pressed

1 large egg, beaten

¼ teaspoon sea salt

⅛ teaspoon ground
  black pepper

Pinch of cayenne pepper

¼ cup (55 g) butter, divided

YIELD: 4 SERVINGS

# SALMON PATTIES WITH LEMON AIOLI

Another one of my favorite meals growing up was my mom's salmon patties. Over the years I've adapted her recipe by removing the grains and made it feel fancier by serving the patties with a lemon aioli sauce.

① To make the aioli: In a small bowl, combine the mayonnaise, lemon juice, horseradish, dill, and pepper. Season to taste with salt. Chill, covered, until ready to serve.

② To make the patties: In a large bowl, add the salmon and break up gently with a fork or wooden spoon. Add the scallion, pepper, mayonnaise, lemon juice, flour, garlic, egg, salt, peppers, and mix until well combined. Divide into 8 equal portions and form into balls; flatten slightly into a 3-inch (7.5 cm) round patty about 1 inch (2.5 cm) thick.

③ Melt 2 tablespoons (28 g) of the butter in a large skillet over medium heat. Fry 4 of the patties for 3 to 4 minutes per side or until golden brown. Remove to a plate and repeat with the remaining 2 tablespoons (28 g) butter and 4 patties.

④ Serve with a dollop of the lemon aioli.

NOTE   The patties can be made ahead and frozen raw. Allow frozen patties to thaw in the refrigerator overnight before panfrying.

# SPAGHETTI AND MEATBALLS

Just because you're eating grain-free doesn't mean you have to give up spaghetti and meatballs. With my grain-free pasta dough, you can roll or extrude it into any shape pasta you desire. It's as easy as following your pasta maker's instructions.

① Preheat the oven to 350°F (180°C, or gas mark 4).

② In a medium skillet over medium heat, melt the fat. Sauté the mushrooms, onion, and garlic until softened, about 2 to 3 minutes.

③ In a food processor, add the cooked vegetables and parsley and pulse to finely chop. Add the beef, pork, Parmesan cheese, egg, salt, and pepper. Pulse until everything is well mixed.

④ Divide the meat mixture into 8 equal portions and roll each into a ball. Set in a casserole dish and bake, uncovered, for 20 minutes or until cooked through to an internal temperature of 160°F (71°C).

⑤ Pour the marinara sauce into a large saucepan over low heat and nestle the cooked meatballs in the sauce.

⑥ Meanwhile, bring a large pot of salted water to a boil over high heat.

⑦ Using a pasta extruder, shape the pasta dough into 12-inch (30 cm)-long spaghetti noodles. Boil for 3 to 5 minutes, or until al dente and then drain. (I recommend tasting it for doneness.)

⑧ Serve the pasta with the marinara sauce, meatballs, and a sprinkle of grated Parmesan cheese.

1 tablespoon (14 g) cooking fat

8 ounces (225 g) white button mushrooms, chopped

1 small onion, finely chopped

1 clove of garlic, pressed or minced

¼ cup (15 g) chopped fresh parsley

8 ounces (225 g) ground beef

8 ounces (225 g) ground pork

¼ cup (25 g) grated Parmesan cheese

1 large egg

½ teaspoon sea salt

¼ teaspoon ground black pepper

4 cups (980 g) marinara sauce

1 recipe for Pasta Dough (page 37)

Grated Parmesan cheese, for garnish

## YIELD: 4 SERVINGS

## MAKE IT A MEAL
Serve with a tossed salad and breadsticks (page 45).

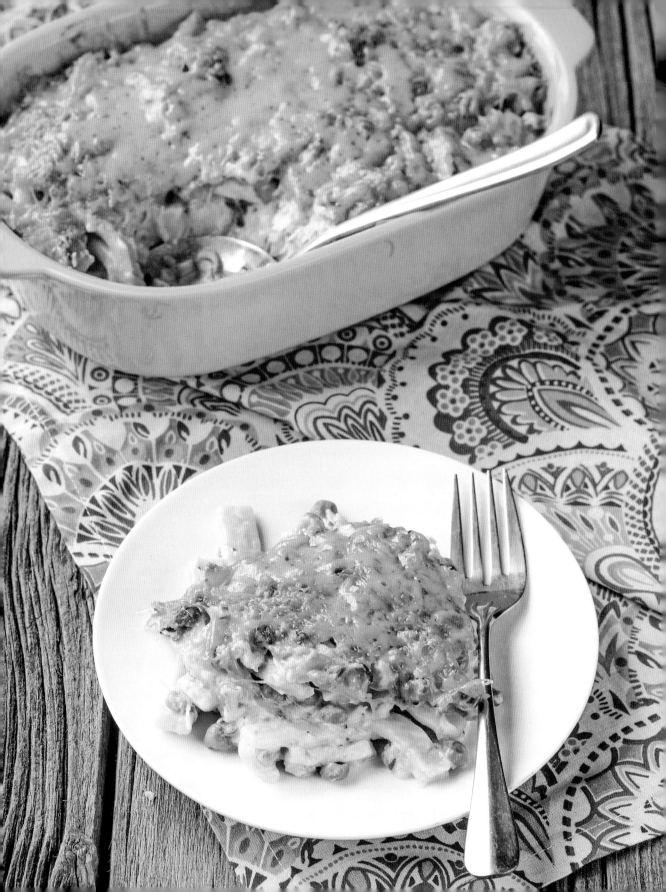

# TUNA NOODLE CASSEROLE

There's no canned soup in this recipe. Mushrooms, onions, celery, and peas all go into this comforting casserole along with homemade noodles (page 37).

① Preheat the oven to 350°F (180°C, or gas mark 4) and grease a 2-quart (2 L) casserole dish.

② Bring a large pot of salted water to a boil.

③ Divide the pasta dough into 2 equal portions. Using additional tapioca starch as needed to avoid sticking, roll out the dough to approximately ¼ inch (6 mm) thick. Use a pizza cutter or knife to cut into noodles approximately ½ x 2 inches (1.3 x 5 cm).

④ Boil the noodles for 7 minutes, drain, and rinse with cold water. Set aside. (The noodles should be al dente.)

⑤ In a large skillet over medium heat, melt the fat. Cook the mushrooms, onion, and garlic until soft, about 3 minutes. Stir in the arrowroot starch. Add the peas, tuna, and 2 tablespoons (10 g) of the Parmesan cheese, mix well, and cook until heated through, about 2 minutes.

⑥ Slowly stir in the half-and-half, heat to a simmer, and cook for 2 to 3 minutes or until slightly thickened. Season with salt and pepper. Remove from the heat and fold in the noodles.

⑦ Transfer the mixture to the prepared casserole dish, cover with foil, and bake for 15 minutes until heated though. Remove from the oven, top with the remaining 2 tablespoons (10 g) Parmesan cheese and the Cheddar cheese, return to the oven, and bake for an additional 5 minutes or until the cheese is melted.

## MAKE IT A MEAL
Serve with a tossed salad.

½ of a recipe for Pasta Dough (page 37)

Tapioca starch

2 tablespoons (28 g) cooking fat

4 ounces (115 g) white button mushrooms, chopped

1 small onion, chopped

1 clove of garlic, pressed or minced

1 tablespoon (11 g) arrowroot starch

1 cup (150 g) fresh or (130 g) frozen peas

12 ounces (340 g) canned tuna, drained

¼ cup (25 g) grated Parmesan cheese, divided

2 cups (475 ml) half-and-half (or 1 cup [235 ml] milk and 1 cup [235 ml] heavy cream)

Sea salt and black pepper, to taste

½ cup (58 g) shredded Cheddar cheese

## YIELD: 4 SERVINGS

1 pound (455 g) baking (russet) potatoes, peeled and cut into 1-inch (2.5 cm) cubes

2 teaspoons butter

1 small onion, finely chopped

8 ounces (225 g) Cheddar cheese, shredded

½ teaspoon sea salt

¼ teaspoon ground black pepper

1 recipe for Pasta Dough (page 37)

Tapioca starch

½ cup (112 g) butter, melted

Optional toppings: sautéed onions and sour cream

YIELD: APPROXIMATELY 20 PIEROGI

# POTATO AND CHEESE PIEROGI

If I could choose a food for my last meal, it would be pierogi. Pierogi are the Polish form of a handmade dumpling. I've made them with my Grammie Elsie since I was a little girl, and I'm excited to share my family recipe—minus the grain. We enjoy them filled with a mixture of mashed potatoes and cheese, dry curd cottage cheese, or sauerkraut. They do take some time to make, but they are so worth it!

(1) Bring a medium saucepan of water to a boil over high heat. Add the potatoes and boil until soft, about 12 to 15 minutes, and then drain.

(2) Meanwhile, in a medium skillet, melt the butter over medium heat. Sauté the onion until translucent, about 4 minutes.

(3) With a hand mixer or stand mixer, combine the potatoes, cheese, and onions. Mix well to combine. Season with the salt and pepper. Allow the potato-cheese mixture to cool completely in the fridge.

(4) Divide the dough into 20 equal portions. Use tapioca starch, as needed, to keep the dough from sticking to the counter or your hands.

## MAKE IT A MEAL

Serve with a tossed salad and steamed broccoli.

⑤ Take a piece of dough and shape it with your fingers into a 3-inch (7.5 cm) round circle. Fill with 2 tablespoons (28 g) of the chilled potato filling. Fold the dough in half around the filling and gently stretch so the edges meet. Pinch and press the edges together to seal.

⑥ Bring a large pot of salted water to a boil. Working in small batches, boil the pierogi for 8 minutes. Scoop out with a slotted spoon, arrange in a single layer on a cookie sheet (with sides), and drizzle with the melted butter. Turn so all are coated well to ensure they do not stick to each other.

⑦ Eat immediately or lightly brown in a skillet over medium heat (using additional butter, as needed). Top with sautéed onions and sour cream, if desired.

NOTE  After the pierogi have been boiled, they can be individually frozen, once cooled, on a baking sheet or plate in a single layer. Once frozen, transfer them to a zip-top plastic bag for up to 6 months. Cook from frozen for best results; do not thaw.

1 pound (455 g) ground beef

1 clove of garlic, pressed or minced

2 cups (230 g) shredded mozzarella cheese, divided

¾ cup (75 g) grated Parmesan cheese, divided

⅓ cup (21 g) chopped fresh parsley

1 large egg

¼ teaspoon sea salt

¼ teaspoon ground black pepper

½ of a recipe for Pasta Dough (page 37)

Tapioca starch

4 cups (980 g) marinara sauce

YIELD: 4 SERVINGS

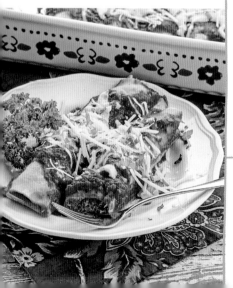

# BAKED MANICOTTI

Using sheets of grain-free pasta dough, you can easily make baked manicotti. Feel free to use the beef mixture in this recipe or substitute your favorite ricotta cheese filling.

① Preheat the oven to 350°F (180°C, or gas mark 4) and grease a 9 x 13-inch (23 x 33 cm) casserole dish.

② In a large skillet over medium heat, brown the beef until cooked through, about 8 minutes. Remove from the heat and allow to cool.

③ In a food processor, combine the beef, garlic, 1 cup (120 g) of the mozzarella cheese, ½ cup (50 g) of the Parmesan cheese, parsley, egg, salt, and pepper. Pulse to combine and chop very finely.

④ Divide the pasta dough into 8 equal portions. Using additional tapioca starch as needed to avoid sticking, roll out each portion to approximately 8 x 4-inch (20 x 10 cm) rectangle, trimming as needed. Spoon one-eighth of the filling mixture 1 inch (2.5 cm) up, along a long edge, and roll up, keeping the filling even as you go along. Place seam-side down in the prepared casserole dish. Repeat with the remaining pasta and filling.

⑤ Pour the marinara sauce over the manicotti, cover, and bake for 20 minutes or until heated through. Remove from the oven and sprinkle the remaining 1 cup (115 g) mozzarella and remaining ¼ cup (25 g) Parmesan over the top and bake, uncovered, for an additional 5 minutes until melted.

## MAKE IT A MEAL
Serve with a tossed salad and a side of spaghetti squash.

# FAJITAS

This is a classic Tex-Mex fajita recipe, complete with strips of skirt steak, onions, and bell peppers—and served sizzling hot with fresh, grain-free tortillas, guacamole, sour cream, and salsa.

① In a small bowl, whisk together the lime juice, cilantro, onion, garlic, cumin, salt, and black pepper and pour into a resealable plastic bag. Add the steak, coat with the marinade, squeeze out excess air, and seal the bag. Marinate in the refrigerator for 4 hours to overnight.

② In a large skillet over medium heat, melt the fat. Remove the beef from the marinade, cook it for 2 minutes, and then add the peppers and sliced onion. Cook until the steak is done to your liking. Serve with warm tortillas and toppings, as desired.

Juice of 1 lime

3 tablespoons (3 g) chopped fresh cilantro

½ of a small onion, finely chopped

1 clove of garlic, pressed or minced

1½ teaspoons ground cumin

1 teaspoon sea salt

½ teaspoon ground black pepper

1 pound (455 g) skirt or sirloin steak, cut into thin strips

2 tablespoons (28 g) cooking fat

1 green bell pepper, cut into strips

1 red bell pepper, cut into strips

1 medium onion, sliced

8 Tortillas (page 41) or Flat Breads (page 40)

Optional toppings: salsa, guacamole, shredded Cheddar cheese, lettuce, tomato, sour cream, or onion

YIELD: 4 SERVINGS

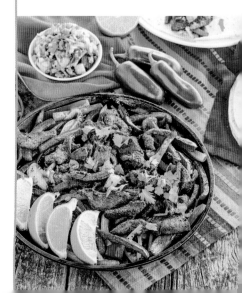

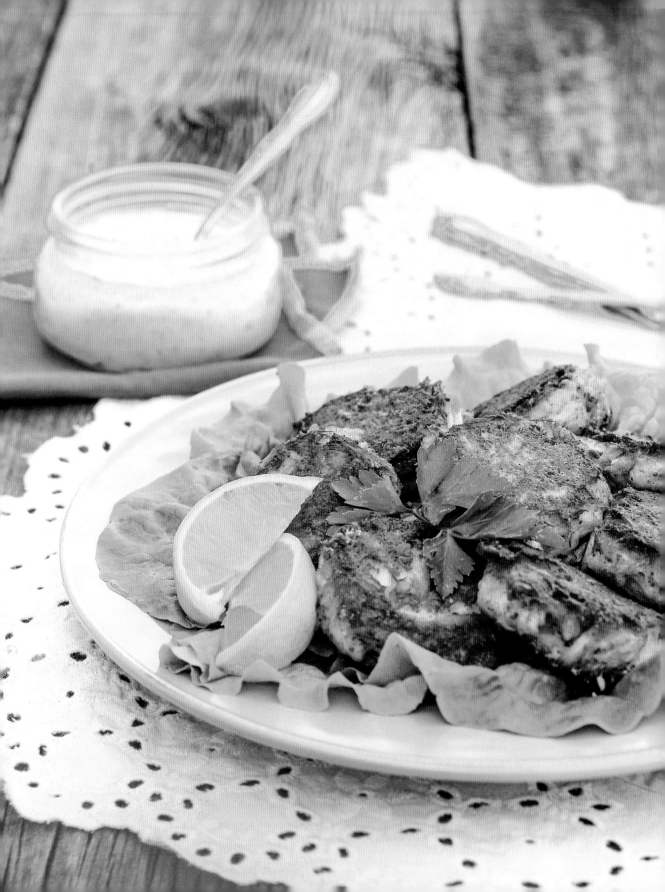

# MARYLAND CRAB CAKES WITH HOMEMADE TARTAR SAUCE

Every June we spend a long weekend at the Lowe's Wharf Marina in Sherwood, Maryland, eating fresh Maryland blue crabs and fishing for striper bass (rockfish). While there, I learned that the key to making an authentic Maryland crab cake is to keep the ingredients simple and avoid overusing binding fillers such as bread and cracker crumbs. Nothing is worse than getting a crab cake that's all filler and hardly any crabmeat! With just a simple swap of ingredients, I've made the perfect crab cake that's jam-packed with delicious crab—use fresh Maryland blue crab if you can find it.

**FOR TARTAR SAUCE:**

½ cup (115 g) mayonnaise

¼ (60 g) cup relish

¼ of a small onion, finely chopped

**FOR CRAB CAKES:**

3 tablespoons (42 g) mayonnaise

1 tablespoon (7 g) coconut flour

1 teaspoon Dijon mustard

1 large egg, beaten

1 teaspoon seafood seasoning, such as Old Bay

1 pound (455 g) fresh or canned lump crabmeat, preferably Maryland blue crab, picked clean of shells

½ cup (112 g) butter, melted

**Lemon wedges, for serving**

YIELD: 4 SERVINGS

① To make the tartar sauce: In a small bowl, combine the mayonnaise, relish, and onion. Store, covered, in the fridge until ready to serve.

② To make the crab cakes: In a large bowl, whisk together the mayonnaise, flour, mustard, egg, and seasoning.

③ Carefully fold in the crabmeat, being as careful as possible not to separate the lumps of meat. Gently form about ½ cup (115 g) of the crab mixture into a cake about 3 inches wide x 1 inch thick (7.5 x 2.5 cm) with your palms. Once formed, set aside on a cookie sheet lined with wax paper. Repeat to form 3 more crab cakes.

④ Heat the butter in a heavy-bottomed skillet over medium-high heat for 2 minutes. Add the crab cakes and fry for about 4 minutes on each side until nice and golden. Transfer to a paper towel–lined plate to drain. Serve with the tartar sauce and plenty of fresh lemon wedges.

NOTE   After you form the crab cakes, they can be frozen on a parchment-lined cookie sheet for approximately 2 hours and then transferred to a sealed container or plastic zip-top bag. Cook frozen cakes just as you would if they were fresh, adding a few minutes of cooking time to each side of the cake.

## FOR GYRO MEAT:

1 pound (455 g) ground beef

1 pound (455 g) ground lamb

2 large eggs

2 tablespoons (14 g) coconut flour

1 tablespoon (8 g) onion powder

1 tablespoon (8 g) garlic powder

1 tablespoon (2 g) dried marjoram

2 teaspoons sea salt

1 teaspoon ground black pepper

½ teaspoon dried oregano

½ teaspoon ground cumin

½ teaspoon dried rosemary

½ teaspoon dried thyme

## FOR TZATZIKI SAUCE:

1 medium English cucumber

1 cup (200 g) Greek yogurt or (230 g) plain whole milk yogurt

1 clove of garlic, minced or pressed

Juice of ½ of a lemon

½ teaspoon dried dill weed

Sea salt and black pepper, to taste

2 recipes for Flat Bread (page 40)

Lettuce, shredded

Tomato, chopped

Onion, chopped

Feta cheese

Yield: 8 servings

# GREEK GYROS WITH TZATZIKI SAUCE

Gyro meat that's typically served in Greek restaurants and at festivals is most often a mixture that contains grains. And gyros are always served on pita bread. You don't need to go without a gyro, just make your own at home.

① To make the gyro meat: In a food processor, combine the beef, lamb, eggs, flour, onion powder, garlic powder, marjoram, salt, pepper, oregano, cumin, rosemary, and thyme. Pulse until well combined. Transfer the mixture to a 4½ x 8½-inch (11.4 x 21.6 cm) loaf pan and firmly press to remove all air pockets. Cover with plastic wrap and refrigerate for 1 to 2 hours to allow the flavors to combine.

② Preheat the oven to 325°F (170°C, or gas mark 3).

③ Line a roasting pan with a damp kitchen towel. Place the loaf pan on the towel, inside the roasting pan, and place in the preheated oven. Pour boiling water into the roasting pan to reach halfway up the sides of the loaf pan.

## MAKE IT A MEAL
Serve with a tossed salad.

④ Bake until the internal temperature registers 160°F (71°C) on a meat thermometer, about 45 minutes to 1 hour. Pour off any accumulated fat, remove the gyro meat from the pan, and allow to cool slightly before slicing thinly.

⑤ To make the tzatziki sauce: Peel and seed the cucumber, and then grate it. Strain and squeeze, using your hands, to remove the excess water from the grated cucumber (you will have ½ to 1 cup [60 to 120 g] of drained, grated cucumber). In a medium bowl, combine the cucumber, yogurt, garlic, lemon juice, and dill. Season with salt and pepper. Chill in the refrigerator until ready to serve.

⑥ Fill each flatbread with several slices of gyro meat, lettuce, tomato, onion, and feta cheese and drizzle with the tzatziki sauce. Fold or roll the flatbread over the fillings (like a taco or burrito).

NOTE   Freeze any leftover gyro meat to use later. Allow to thaw in the refrigerator and then reheat.

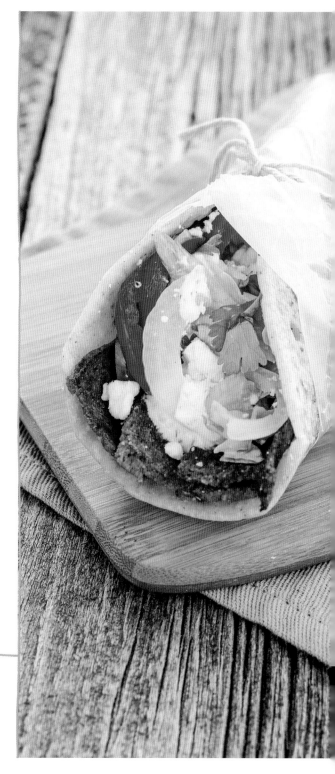

1 pound (455 g) ground beef

1 tablespoon (8 g) chili powder

1 teaspoon onion powder

1 teaspoon garlic powder

½ teaspoon sea salt

½ teaspoon paprika

¼ teaspoon cumin

⅛ teaspoon crushed red pepper

2 recipes for Tortillas (page 41)

Optional toppings: salsa, guacamole, shredded Cheddar cheese, lettuce, tomato, sour cream, or onion

YIELD: 4 SERVINGS

# CRISPY BEEF TACOS

Just because you've given up grains doesn't mean you can't have tacos, the kind that yield a satisfying crunch when you bite into them. Don't feel limited to just the fillings I've included in this recipe; feel free to fill your tacos with anything you like! We love using leftover battered fish (page 143) to make fish tacos with Homemade Tartar Sauce (page 143).

① Preheat the oven to 350°F (180°C, or gas mark 4).

② In a large skillet over medium heat, sauté the ground beef with the spices until cooked through, about 8 minutes.

③ Meanwhile, make the tortillas according to the recipe. Once cooked (but soft), gently bend or fold the tortillas to go over 1 or 2 of the bars of an oven rack, making a taco shell that is pointing down. Bake for 5 minutes or until crispy.

④ Fill the crispy taco shells with seasoned ground beef and toppings, as desired.

## MAKE IT A MEAL
Serve with Cauliflower Rice (page 35).

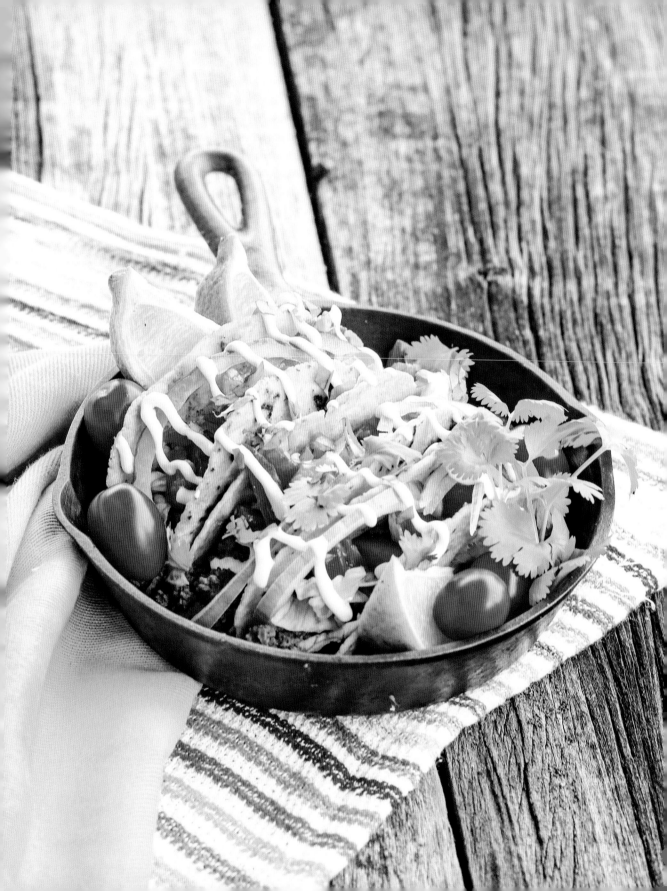

1 pound (455 g) boneless, skinless chicken breast or thighs

2 teaspoons garam masala, divided

½ teaspoon sea salt

Pinch of cayenne pepper

3 tablespoons (42 g) butter, divided

1 small onion, chopped

2 cloves of garlic, minced or pressed

2 teaspoons freshly grated ginger

Juice of ½ of a lemon

1 teaspoon cumin

1 teaspoon chili powder

1 bay leaf

¼ teaspoon ground fenugreek

⅛ teaspoon ground coriander

1 cup (250 g) tomato puree

1 cup (235 ml) half-and-half (or ½ cup [120 ml] heavy cream and ½ cup [120 ml] milk)

½ cup (70 g) raw cashews (unsalted)

¼ cup (60 g) plain whole milk yogurt

Black pepper, to taste

YIELD: 4 SERVINGS

# INDIAN BUTTER CHICKEN

Indian butter chicken (chicken makhani) is one of my favorite Indian dishes. Though traditionally it does not contain grains, many people take a shortcut and use flour to thicken the sauce, and it's frequently served with rice and grain-containing naan or chapatis. Unless you are certain of the ingredients, it's best to make it yourself. This is a full-flavored dish that can be made as mild or spicy as you wish by adjusting the cayenne pepper. Serve with Cauliflower Rice (page 35) and Flat Bread (page 40).

① Cut the chicken into bite-size pieces and season with 1 teaspoon of the garam masala and the salt and pepper.

② Heat 1 tablespoon (14 g) of the butter in a large heavy skillet over medium heat. Cook the chicken until lightly browned on all sides, about 10 minutes. Remove from the pan and set aside.

③ Return the skillet to medium heat and add the remaining 2 tablespoons (28 g) butter. When melted, add the onion, garlic, and ginger and sauté until soft, about 3 to 4 minutes. Stir in the lemon juice, remaining 1 teaspoon of garam masala, cumin, chili powder, bay leaf, fenugreek, and coriander. Cook, stirring, for 1 minute. Add the tomato puree, reduce the heat, and simmer for about 5 minutes, stirring frequently.

④ Remove the bay leaf and then transfer the sauce to a blender, along with the half-and-half, cashews, and yogurt. Carefully puree until the sauce is completely smooth.

⑤ Reduce the heat to low, add the reserved cooked chicken and sauce back to the skillet, and simmer for 10 minutes, stirring frequently. Season to taste with salt and pepper.

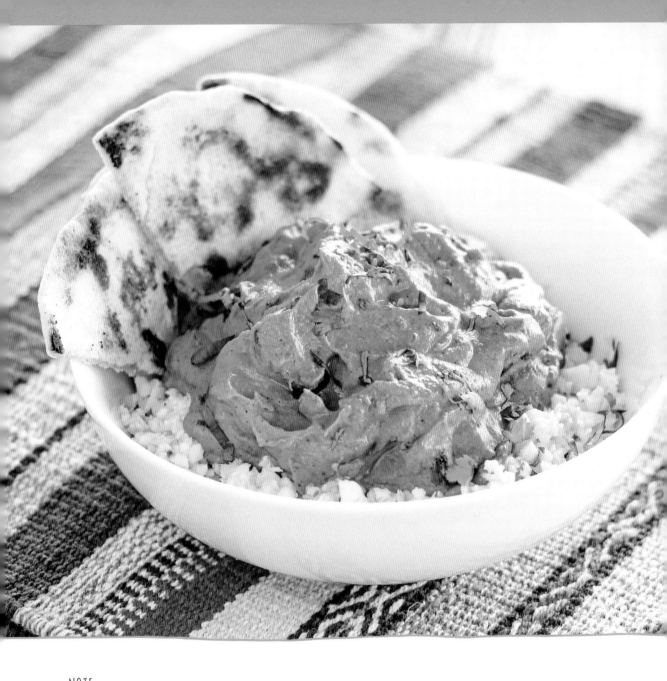

NOTE  Fenugreek (whole or ground seeds) is used in Middle Eastern and Indian cooking. It can be found in the spice section of most grocery stores.

1 can (14 ounces, or 390 g) coconut milk

2 tablespoons (30 g) Thai red curry paste

1 tablespoon (12 g) coconut sugar

1 pound (455 g) wild-caught shrimp, peeled and deveined

4 cups (approximately 480 g total) assorted vegetables (onions, carrot, broccoli, bell peppers, mushrooms, zucchini, etc.), cut into bite-size pieces

Fish sauce

Sea salt and black pepper, to taste

YIELD: 4 SERVINGS

# THAI RED CURRY SHRIMP

Like Indian Butter Chicken (page 148), this dish isn't traditionally made with grains, but it is frequently served with rice (grain). This is the quickest and easiest Thai red curry recipe ever. It's great for an impressive dinner party because it tastes delicious but hardly takes any time to make.

① In a large skillet over medium heat, combine the coconut milk, Thai red curry paste, and coconut sugar. Whisk or stir well and simmer for 5 minutes.

② Add the shrimp and vegetables and stir until coated with the sauce. Simmer until the shrimp are cooked (no longer pink) and the veggies are crisp-tender. Season with a few drops of fish sauce, salt, and pepper.

## MAKE IT A MEAL
Serve with 4 cups (400 g) cooked Cauliflower Rice (page 35).

NOTE  Although there isn't much fish sauce used in this dish, it is definitely worth adding. See page 199 for my recommendations on which fish sauce to buy.

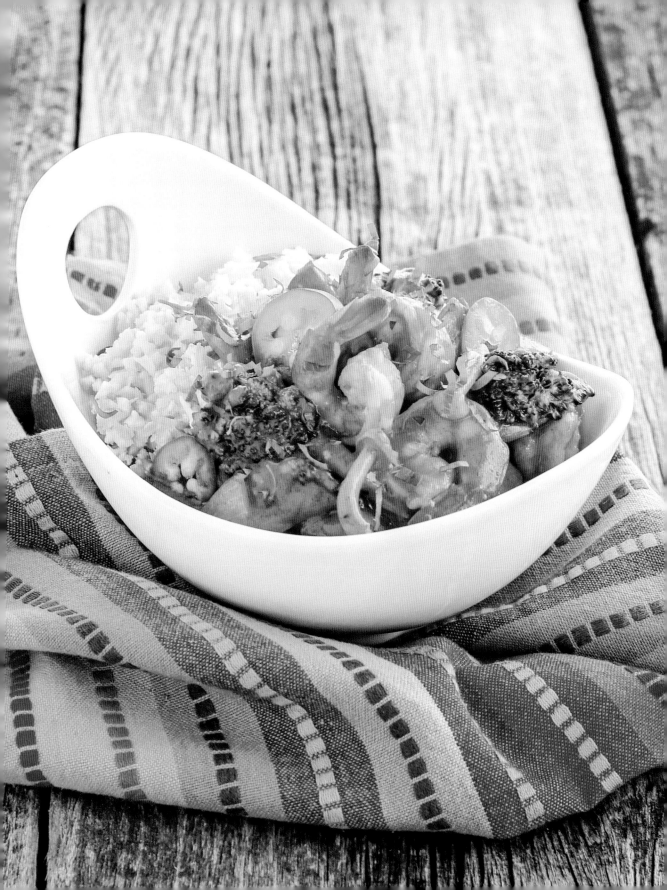

- 1¾ cups (210 g) tapioca starch, plus additional for dusting
- ¼ cup (48 g) potato starch
- ¼ cup (12 g) nutritional yeast flakes
- ¾ teaspoon sea salt
- ¾ teaspoon Italian seasoning
- ¾ teaspoon garlic powder
- ¼ teaspoon white pepper
- ½ cup (120 ml) half-and-half (or ¼ cup [60 ml] heavy cream and ¼ cup [60 ml] milk)
- 2 tablespoons (28 g) cooking fat, melted
- 1 large egg, beaten
- Toppings: pizza sauce, cheese, pepperoni, etc.

Yield: One 16-inch (40 cm) thin crust pizza

# NEW YORK-STYLE PIZZA

The key to a really good pizza is, of course, the crust. We make grain-free pizza at our house at least twice a month, so you can be sure this recipe comes to you after years of kitchen testing! Also, the fact that this dough comes together in just a few minutes and doesn't need time to rise means that we can have pizza for dinner any night of the week.

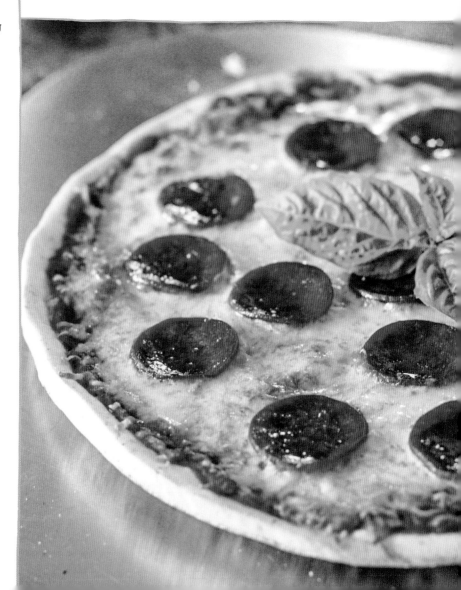

(1) Preheat the oven to 450°F (230°C, or gas mark 8). Line a pizza pan or baking sheet with parchment paper.

(2) In a large bowl, whisk together the starches, nutritional yeast, salt, Italian seasoning, garlic powder, and pepper.

(3) In a separate small bowl or measuring cup, whisk together the half-and-half, fat, and egg. Add the liquid ingredients to the dry ingredients and stir to combine. The mixture will resemble a firm dough (add more tapioca starch if the dough is too wet).

(4) Using your fingers, lightly dusted with additional tapioca starch, press the dough into a 16-inch (40 cm) circle on the pizza pan or baking sheet. Bake the plain crust for 10 minutes or until crispy. Remove the baked crust from the oven and top as desired.

(5) Return the pizza to the oven and bake for an additional 10 to 15 minutes or until the toppings are hot and bubbling. Allow to cool briefly before slicing.

## MAKE IT A MEAL

Serve with a large tossed salad.

NOTES  To use a pizza or baking stone, preheat the stone in the oven. Prepare the crust on parchment paper and transfer it to your preheated stone to bake, according to the recipe. The dough can be divided into individual-size pizza crusts, instead of one large crust. Baked crusts can be frozen for up to 6 months; no need to thaw before topping and baking. Nutritional yeast can be found as flakes or powder in the bulk foods aisle of most natural food stores or online (see Resources, page 199). It has a strong flavor that can be described as nutty, cheesy, or creamy. Do not confuse it with brewer's yeast, as they cannot be used interchangeably.

**FOR MARINADE:**

1 egg white

3 tablespoons (45 ml) coconut aminos

3 tablespoons (45 ml) dry sherry

3 tablespoons (33 g) arrowroot starch

¼ teaspoon baking soda

1 pound (455 g) boneless, skinless chicken breast and/or thighs, cut into bite-size pieces

**FOR BREADING:**

1 cup (120 g) tapioca starch

½ cup (56 g) blanched almond flour

½ teaspoon sea salt

½ teaspoon garlic powder

½ teaspoon onion powder

Pinch of crushed red pepper flakes

**FOR SAUCE:**

4 tablespoons (48 g) cane sugar

3 tablespoons (45 ml) coconut aminos

3 tablespoons (45 ml) chicken broth/stock (page 93)

2 tablespoons (28 ml) dry sherry

2 tablespoons (28 ml) apple cider vinegar

1 tablespoon (11 g) arrowroot starch

1 teaspoon toasted sesame oil

# GENERAL TSO'S CHICKEN

General Tso's chicken is a sweet, slightly spicy, deep-fried chicken dish that is popularly served in American Chinese restaurants. If you are sensitive to spicy foods, feel free to leave out the red chiles completely for a milder version of this recipe.

This recipe isn't the quickest one in this book to make, but I promise you it is completely worth the extra effort to achieve the taste and texture you've been craving. There are no special techniques—just several simple steps—to bring everything together.

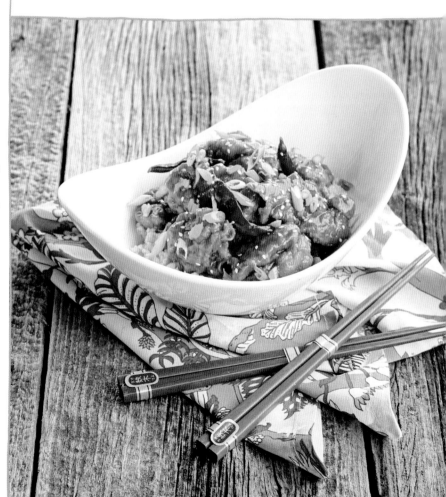

1. To make the marinade: Beat the egg white in a large bowl until frothy. Add the coconut aminos and sherry and whisk to combine. Whisk in the arrowroot starch and baking soda. Add the chicken and mix well to coat. Cover with plastic wrap and refrigerate for at least 30 minutes and up to 24 hours.

2. To make the breading: In a large bowl, combine the starch, flour, salt, garlic powder, onion powder, and pepper. Set aside.

3. To make the sauce: In a small bowl, whisk together the sugar, coconut aminos, broth, sherry, vinegar, arrowroot, and oil. Whisk well to remove all lumps. Set aside.

4. In a large skillet over medium heat, combine the fat, garlic, ginger, scallion, and chiles, if using. Cook, stirring, until the vegetables are aromatic and soft, but not browned, about 3 minutes.

5. Stir the sauce mixture and add to the skillet, making sure to mix well (it can separate). Cook, stirring, until the sauce boils and thickens, about 1 minute. Remove from the heat and stir in the scallions.

6. Remove the chicken from the marinade and toss in the breading mixture (do not discard the marinade). Remove the chicken from the breading mixture and set aside. Take each piece of chicken, dip it back into the marinade, and then coat it with the breading again (marinade-dry-marinade-dry). Place the breaded chicken pieces in a single layer on a wax paper–lined plate and put in the refrigerator for at least 30 minutes.

7. Heat the fat in a large wok or Dutch oven to 350°F (180°C).

8. Carefully place the chicken into the hot oil and fry until cooked through and very crispy, about 4 minutes. Transfer the chicken to a paper towel–lined plate to drain.

9. Meanwhile, return the sauce to a simmer over medium heat. Fold the chicken into the sauce, making sure all pieces are coated well. Serve immediately.

**2 teaspoons cooking fat**

**2 cloves of garlic, pressed or minced**

**2 teaspoons minced fresh ginger**

**2 teaspoons minced scallion bottoms (white part only, about 1 scallion)**

**8 small dried Thai red chiles or other dried red chiles (optional)**

**6 scallions, sliced diagonally**

**6 cups (1.4 kg) lard or palm oil, for frying**

## YIELD: 4 SERVINGS

## MAKE IT A MEAL
Serve with cooked Cauliflower Rice (page 35) and/or steamed broccoli.

½ cup (96 g) cane sugar

½ cup (120 ml) water

½ cup (50 g) walnuts

¼ cup (60 g) mayonnaise

2 tablespoons (40 g) honey

1 tablespoon (15 ml) sweetened condensed milk

3 large egg whites

½ cup (64 g) arrowroot starch

1 cup (225 g) lard, palm oil, or coconut oil, for frying

1 pound (455 g) wild-caught large-size shrimp, peeled and deveined

YIELD: 4 SERVINGS

# HONEY WALNUT SHRIMP

Budget-friendly crispy battered shrimp tossed in a creamy, sweet mayonnaise mixture, topped with caramelized walnuts. What's not to love about that?

① In a small saucepan, stir together the sugar and water. Bring to a boil and add the walnuts. Boil for 2 minutes, then drain and spread the walnuts on a cookie sheet to dry.

② In a medium bowl, stir together the mayonnaise, honey, and sweetened condensed milk. Set aside.

③ Whip the egg whites in a medium bowl until foamy. Stir in the arrowroot starch until it has a pasty consistency.

④ Heat the oil in a heavy, deep skillet over medium-high heat. Dip the shrimp into the egg batter and then fry in the hot oil until golden brown, about 5 minutes. Remove with a slotted spoon and drain on paper towels. Toss the cooked shrimp to coat in the sauce and sprinkle the candied walnuts on top.

## MAKE IT A MEAL
Serve with a side of steamed broccoli or Egg Rolls (page 80).

# HAM AND SHRIMP FRIED RICE

This restaurant-style fried rice tastes just like the fried rice you would find at your favorite Chinese restaurant—only it's made grain-free by using Cauliflower Rice (page 35).

① In a skillet over medium heat, scramble the eggs in 1 tablespoon (14 g) of the cooking fat until cooked through, about 3 to 5 minutes. Use a spatula to coarsely chop the cooked eggs into bite-size pieces and set aside.

② In a large skillet over medium heat, melt the remaining 3 tablespoons (42 g) fat. Cook the ham, shrimp, onion, celery, mushrooms, and coconut aminos until the shrimp are cooked through (no longer pink), about 3 to 5 minutes.

③ Stir in the carrot, broccoli, peas, cabbage, and cauliflower rice. Cook until all the veggies are lightly cooked and crisp-tender, about 2 to 3 minutes. Season with additional coconut aminos, to taste, if desired.

④ Just before serving, toss in the scrambled egg.

4 large eggs, beaten

¼ cup (55 g) cooking fat, divided

1 cup (150 g) diced uncured ham

8 ounces (225 g) wild-caught shrimp, peeled and deveined

1 small onion, chopped

1 rib of celery, chopped

4 ounces (115 g) mushrooms

¼ cup (60 ml) coconut aminos, plus more to taste

½ of a carrot, grated

½ cup (36 g) broccoli florets

1 cup peas, (150 g) fresh or (130 g) frozen

3 cups (225 g) shredded napa cabbage (½ of a medium head)

4 cups (400 g) raw Cauliflower Rice (page 35)

## YIELD: 4 SERVINGS

## MAKE IT A MEAL
Serve with Egg Rolls (page 80).

# Chapter 8:

# KID-APPROVED RECIPES

AS YOU MIGHT IMAGINE, my family talks a lot about food and cooking. And it's not just because I love to cook or even that it's part of my job. We talk about it because understanding nutrition is an important foundation for building a healthy life. As an extension, teaching children where their food comes from and how to prepare it in a healthy way is a gift that will benefit them for their entire lives.

One of the saddest problems today is the increasing number of obese and overweight children. In the United States, childhood obesity has increased more than threefold in past thirty-five years. It's a common misconception that as long as you're active or going to the gym on a regular basis, you can slack a little on your diet. That is 100 percent not the case. You can't outrun bad eating habits and neither can your kids.

Healthy (and unhealthy) eating habits are first established in the home. Family meals, parental eating and cooking practices, and home availability of healthful foods have all been associated with the establishment and mainte-nance of healthy eating habits. Children will mimic parents in their consumption of fruit and vegetables, as indicated by a recent review in *Health Education Research*. And those healthy eating habits will serve children well as they grow, establishing patterns that will influence their health well into adulthood.

But is it safe for children to eat grain-free?

Both babies and children evolved eating a grain-free diet, the same as adult humans did for thousands of years. Our ancestors fed their little ones a healthy, nutrient-rich diet without any processed or packaged foods, soy formula, crackers, or rice cereal. In the book *Nutrition and Physical Degeneration*, Weston A. Price notes that traditional (and very healthy) people all over the world have given their children the same whole foods they themselves eat from the very start of life.

My friends Stacy and Matt share their family's amazing story of transformation—attributed to changing the way that they eat, eliminating grains, and eating more real foods—at PaleoParents.com and in their book *Eat Like a Dinosaur*. After going Paleo, Stacy and Matt both lost a significant amount of weight and their health improved, but they saw the most amazing impact in their children. By simply changing their diet, their two sons (ages three and five at the time) no longer suffered from behavioral and self-control issues, attention-deficit disorder, asthma, allergies, and eczema. Their son Cole went from being nearly expelled for bad behavior to being one of the best behaved in his class!

Although children aren't interested in learning about how and why grains in their food affect their health, they are eager to eat all the foods they've grown accustomed to enjoying. If you're switching your children to a grain-free diet, providing them with their favorite foods—only made without grains—will enable them to reap the benefits of a healthier diet without the struggles of changing their familiar way of eating. With foods such as Chicken Tenders (page 160), Soft Pretzels (page 164), and Pepperoni Rolls (page 161), your kids won't even notice they're eating healthier!

Many of the recipes in this chapter can be doubled or even tripled and made ahead to be packed into lunches along with raw veggies, cheese cubes, and fruit. Using supplies such as stainless insulated thermoses and stainless steel lunch containers makes it easy to pack leftovers and less-traditional lunch foods. They are dishwasher safe, leakproof, and won't leach BPA or other chemicals into their food. Getting your children involved in preparing their lunches will also get them excited to eat the lunch they've helped prepare, rather than trading it for less-healthy options.

Because we don't have children of our own, I reached out to the experts for help. Our friends' children were more than willing to give me the scoop on their favorite foods and give the final thumbs-up on my grain-free recipes.

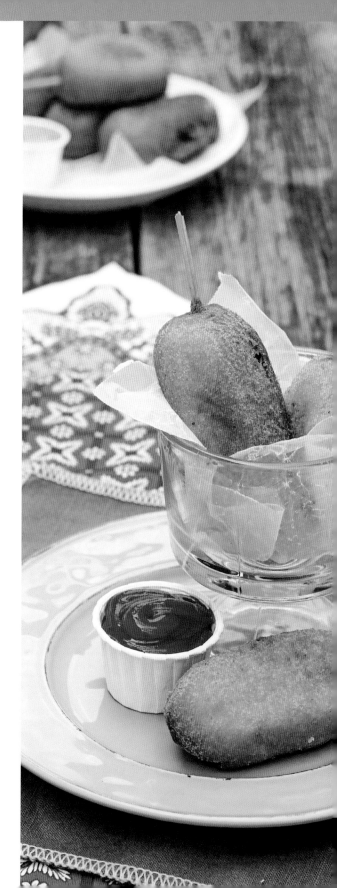

1½ cups (150 g) grated
   Parmesan cheese

½ teaspoon garlic powder

½ teaspoon Italian seasoning

1 pound (455 g) chicken
   breast tenders

2 large eggs

YIELD: 4 SERVINGS

# CHICKEN TENDERS

It doesn't get much easier than coating chicken tenders with a Parmesan cheese breading and baking until crispy. They are also delicious made ahead and packed in school lunches. Either way, serve with a side of tomato sauce, if desired.

①  Preheat the oven to 400°F (200°C, or gas mark 6) and line a baking sheet with parchment paper.

②  Combine the Parmesan cheese, garlic powder, and Italian seasoning in a shallow dish. Beat the eggs in a separate shallow dish.

③  Dip the chicken tenders into the beaten eggs and then into the seasoned Parmesan mixture, using your hands to press the cheese firmly onto the chicken.

④  Arrange the chicken tenders on the prepared baking sheet so that they are not touching. Bake for 10 minutes, turn them over, and bake for an additional 10 minutes or until the chicken is cooked through and the cheese breading is browned and crispy. Serve warm.

NOTE   Breaded tenders can be refrigerated for up to 2 days or frozen for up to 3 months, prior to baking. Do not thaw frozen tenders before baking and extend cooking times by 5 to 7 minutes on each side to ensure they are cooked through and crispy.

# PEPPERONI ROLLS

The pepperoni roll is a snack popular in West Virginia and nearby western Pennsylvania, Maryland, and Ohio. We live 15 minutes north of West Virginia—where the roll is ubiquitous, particularly in convenience stores, and is arguably the food most closely associated with the state. Great for lunches or when traveling, and served warm or cold with tomato sauce, they are always a kid-approved snack.

1 cup (128 g) arrowroot starch

2 cups (225 g) shredded Cheddar cheese

1 teaspoon garlic powder

1 teaspoon onion powder

1 teaspoon sea salt

¼ teaspoon white pepper

1 tablespoon (8 g) baking powder (page 20)

2 large eggs

4 ounces (115 g) uncured pepperoni, sliced

½ cup (60 g) shredded mozzarella cheese

¼ cup (25 g) shredded Parmesan cheese

**Yield: 8 pepperoni rolls**

① Preheat the oven to 325°F (170°C, or gas mark 3) and line a baking sheet with parchment paper.

② In a food processor, combine the starch, cheese, powders, salt, pepper, and baking powder. Process on high until there are no large, noticeable shreds of cheese left. Add the eggs and pulse until it forms a dough.

③ Divide the dough into 8 equal portions. Roll or press each portion into an oval approximately 8 x 4 inches (20 x 10 cm). Layer approximately ½ ounce (15 g) of the sliced pepperoni on the dough, leaving about ¼ inch (6 mm) around the edges, and roll up.

④ Place the pepperoni rolls, seam-side down, on the baking sheet so that they are not touching and bake for 15 minutes. Remove from the oven and top each with the mozzarella and Parmesan cheeses. Return to the oven and bake for an additional 5 minutes.

⑤ Transfer to a wire rack and allow to cool slightly.

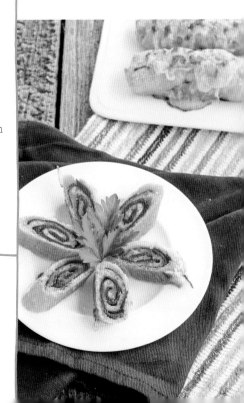

NOTE   Cooked and cooled pepperoni rolls can be stored in the refrigerator for up to a week or frozen for up to 6 months and reheated in the oven at 325°F (170°C, or gas mark 3).

1 cup (112 g) blanched almond flour

½ cup (60 g) tapioca starch

½ cup (64 g) arrowroot starch

2 teaspoons baking powder (page 20)

2 tablespoons (40 g) honey

¼ teaspoon sea salt

3 large eggs

¼ cup (55 g) cooking fat, melted

1 teaspoon apple cider vinegar

6 or 8 uncured hot dogs

Optional: lard or palm oil, for frying

## YIELD: 16 CORN DOGS OR 12 MUFFINS

NOTES Both corn dogs and muffins can be frozen in an airtight container for up to 6 months. Reheat from frozen in a 350°F (180°C, or gas mark 4) oven until hot. The batter can also be used without hot dogs to make No-Corn, Cornbread Muffins.

# NO-CORN, CORN DOG

This batter mixture has all the flavor of cornbread, even though there are no grains included. If you'd like to skip the deep-frying, or if you don't have bamboo skewers on hand, this recipe easily converts to baked muffins. Serve with ketchup, mustard, and/or Cheese Sauce (page 42).

① In a blender, combine the flour, starches, baking powder, honey, salt, eggs, fat, and vinegar. Blend on high for 30 seconds.

② *Deep-Fried Dogs:* Cut 8 hot dogs in half and push each onto half of a bamboo skewer, leaving about 2 inches (5 cm) of the skewer exposed. Fill the deep fryer or a large heavy-bottomed pot with 2 inches (5 cm) of fat and heat to 325°F (170°C).

③ Working with 1 hot dog at a time, using the skewer as a handle, remove any moisture from the hot dog with a paper towel and then dip into the batter mixture, coating well. Allow extra batter to drip off, but leave the hot dog completely coated.

④ Carefully place the battered hot dog into the hot fat and fry until golden brown on all sides, turning as necessary. Remove the corn dogs from the fat by using metal tongs to pick up the exposed skewer and allow to drain on a paper towel–lined plate.

⑤ *Baked Muffins:* Preheat the oven to 350°F (180°C, or gas mark 4) and grease a 12-cup muffin pan. Cut 6 hot dogs in half.

⑥ Pour just enough batter into each muffin cup to thinly cover the bottom, top with a piece of hot dog, and then pour additional batter over the hot dog to cover.

⑦ Bake for 15 to 20 minutes or until a toothpick inserted into the side of a muffin comes out clean. Remove and transfer to a cooling rack.

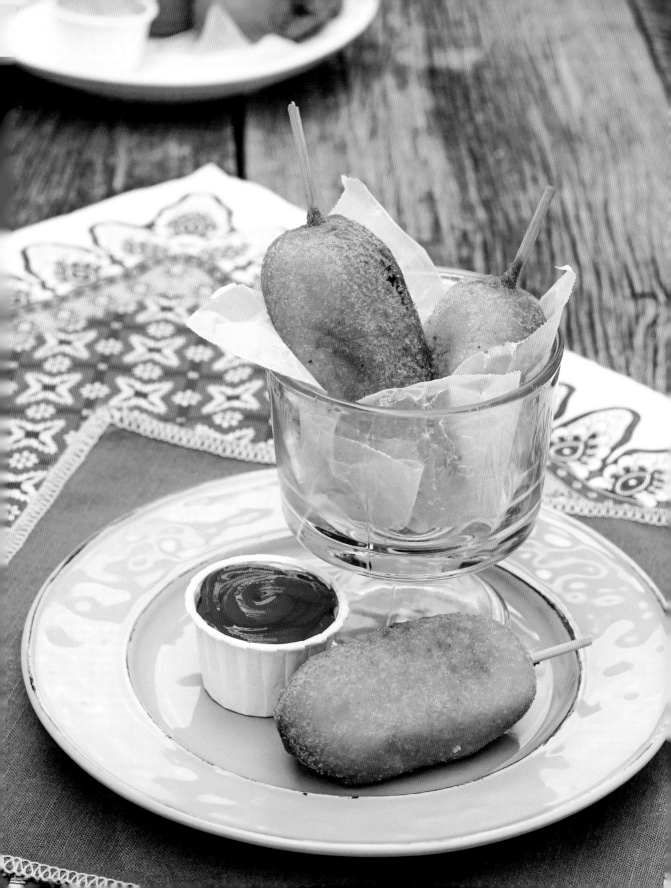

**FOR PRETZELS:**

1¼ cups (285 ml) warm water, 100° to 110°F (38° to 43°C)

1 tablespoon (20 g) honey

1 packet (2¼ teaspoons, or 7 g) active dry yeast

2 cups (224 g) blanched almond flour

1 cup (128 g) arrowroot starch

1 cup (120 g) tapioca starch, plus more for dusting

1 teaspoon sea salt

1 teaspoon baking powder (page 20)

¼ cup (50 g) cooking fat, melted

**FOR BAKING SODA BATH:**

8 to 10 cups (1.9 to 2.4 L) water

½ cup (110 g) baking soda

**FOR TOPPING:**

1 large egg yolk

1 teaspoon honey

Sea salt

Mustard or Cheese Sauce (page 42), for serving (optional)

## Yield: 12 soft pretzels

# SOFT PRETZELS

These warm and buttery, grain-free homemade soft pretzels can be topped with sea salt for a savory snack or cinnamon and sugar for a sweet treat.

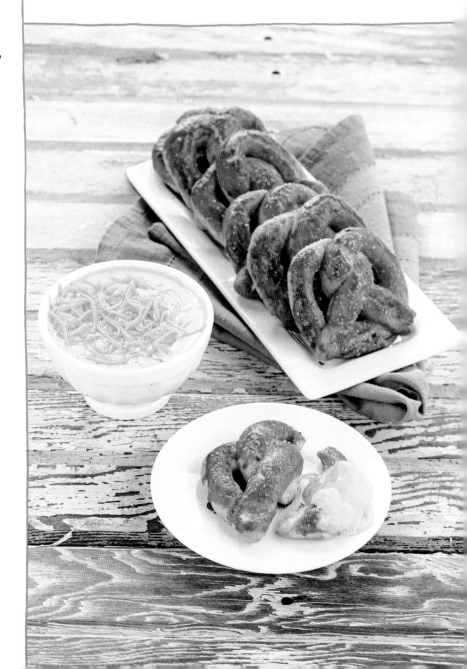

(1) To make the pretzels: In a small bowl, whisk together the water, honey, and yeast. Allow to sit for 5 to 10 minutes until the mixture foams.

(2) In the bowl of a stand mixer, combine the flour, starches, salt, and baking powder. Mix well. Add the fat and the yeast mixture. With the dough hook, mix on medium speed until the dough comes together, scraping the sides and bottom of the bowl as needed.

(3) Once combined fully, continue to mix on high speed for 2 minutes. The dough should be slightly tacky, but not too wet so it doesn't come together and hold.

(4) Turn the oven to 350°F (180°C, or gas mark 4) for exactly 2 minutes and then turn off the heat (this will create a warm oven for the dough to rise in). Loosely cover the bowl of dough with plastic wrap and place in the warmed oven. Allow the dough to rise for 45 minutes, undisturbed.

(5) Turn the dough out onto a work surface lightly dusted with tapioca starch. Using a sharp knife, divide the dough carefully into 12 equal portions. Roll each piece into a 12-inch (30 cm) log and then twist into a pretzel shape, pressing to seal down the ends. Place the pretzels on a parchment-lined baking sheet, 2 inches (5 cm) apart. (You may need 2 baking sheets.)

(6) Heat the oven (again) to 350°F (180°C, or gas mark 4) for exactly 2 minutes and then turn off the heat. Place the pretzels (uncovered) in the warmed oven. Allow the pretzels to rise again for 45 minutes, undisturbed.

(7) Remove the risen pretzels from the oven and preheat the oven to 450°F (230°C, or gas mark 8).

(8) To make the baking soda bath: In a large pot over high heat, bring the water and baking soda just to a boil. Once the water comes to a boil, reduce the heat so that the water is gently simmering. A full rolling boil will damage the pretzels.

(9) Working in small batches, carefully place a few pretzels into the baking soda bath. Simmer for about 30 seconds, gently turn over the pretzels, and simmer for an additional 30 seconds. Remove the pretzels from the bath using a slotted spoon and place them back onto the parchment-lined baking sheet. Repeat until all the pretzels are done.

(10) To make the topping: Whisk together the egg yolk and honey, gently brush on each pretzel, and sprinkle with salt.

(11) Place the pretzels in the center of the oven and bake until golden brown all over, about 20 minutes. Let cool on the baking sheet for a few minutes before transferring to cooling racks. Serve warm with mustard, if desired.

NOTES   Pretzels can be stored at room temperature in an airtight container and reheated in the oven.

For cinnamon sugar–topped pretzels, combine ¼ cup (50 g) cane sugar with 2 tablespoons (14 g) cinnamon and sprinkle on the pretzels instead of sea salt.

8 uncured hot dogs

½ cup (64 g) arrowroot starch

1 cup (115 g) shredded provolone cheese

1½ teaspoons baking powder (page 20)

¼ teaspoon garlic powder

¼ teaspoon onion powder

¼ teaspoon sea salt

⅛ teaspoon white pepper

1 large egg

Optional: ketchup and/or mustard, for dipping

## Yield: 16 weenie tots

# WEENIE TOTS

When we first moved into our house, we had parties for every Pittsburgh Steelers game, and one of our standard appetizers were Weenie Tots made with refrigerated crescent roll dough. As the years have passed, we've made our parties healthier, but the menu hasn't changed much since I've learned how to adapt our favorite recipes to be grain-free!

① Preheat the oven to 325°F (170°C, or gas mark 3) and line a baking sheet with parchment paper. Cut the hot dogs in half and set aside.

② In a food processor, combine the arrowroot starch, cheese, baking powder, and seasonings. Process on high until there are no large, noticeable shreds of cheese left. Add the egg and pulse until it forms a dough.

③ Divide the dough into 16 equal portions. Roll out each portion into a 4- to 6-inch (10 to 15 cm) log and wrap in a spiral around a hot dog half.

④ Arrange on the baking sheet so that they are not touching and bake for 15 minutes until the dough is firm and lightly brown.

⑤ Transfer to a wire rack and allow to cool slightly. Serve with ketchup and/or mustard, as desired.

NOTE   Tots can be stored in the refrigerator for up to a week or frozen for up to 6 months and reheated in a 325°F (170°C, or gas mark 3) oven.

# HAM AND CHEESE "HOT POCKET"

Using my grain-free Flat Bread (page 40), you can make a variety of hot pockets, such as pepperoni and cheese; chicken, broccoli and Cheddar; and even corned beef, Swiss cheese, and sauerkraut. And I always make a few filled with leftover Sloppy Joe (page 115) mixture.

1 recipe for Flat Bread (page 40)

8 ounces (225 g) uncured, sliced deli ham

1 cup (115 g) shredded Cheddar cheese

YIELD: 4 HOT POCKETS

① Preheat the oven to 350°F (180°C, or gas mark 4). Line a baking sheet with parchment paper.

② Make the flat breads and cook them in the skillet according to the recipe, but do not bake them.

③ Fill each of the flat breads with one-fourth of the ham and one-fourth of the cheese. Fold in half and, using a fork and firm pressure, seal the open edges (it will make a half-moon). Set on the baking sheet.

④ Bake for 15 minutes or until crispy. Let cool slightly on a wire rack.

NOTE   Baked hot pockets can be indivdually wrapped in plastic bags and frozen for quick meals. Reheat in a 350°F (180°C, or gas mark 4) oven for 15 to 20 minutes or until heated through.

# Chapter 9:

# DESSERTS, SWEETS, AND TREATS

IF YOU'RE INTIMIDATED by baking, then I have good news for you: grain-free ingredients take all the stress out of the baking process. You don't need to worry about ruining a recipe by overmixing, deciphering complicated ingredients, or following a long list of steps. Most grain-free baking recipes can be made quickly, with just a few minutes in a blender, food processor, or mixer before being poured into a pan. From cookies to cakes, these recipes are all so simple and taste so great that no one will guess they're grain-free!

With just a few grain-free baking ingredients stocked in your pantry (see chapter 2), you'll be prepared to try out any of these delicious recipes. But because this chapter is all about sweets, here's a list of my preferred sweeteners.

**Cane sugar:** Unrefined cane sugar is a better choice than white sugar because it has not had all the beneficial minerals stripped away. Unrefined cane sugar can be substituted in most recipes 1:1 for white sugar.

**Stevia:** *Stevia rebaudiana* is a perennial shrub that is native to Paraguay and Brazil. Stevia contains intensely sweet compounds, and it has long been used as a sugar substitute in Japan, China, and South America. I don't use it often when baking, but I do enjoy it as a sweetener in iced teas and coffee. If you choose stevia, make sure it is a whole-leaf product and does not contain the processed product rebaudioside A.

**Maple syrup** is a traditional and whole sweetener that has consistently played an integral part in the economies of North America ever since Native Americans first taught the early European settlers how to tap maple trees and boil down the sap. The darker, more flavorful "grade B" contains higher concentrations of minerals and phytochemicals and is considered the healthiest maple syrup on the market.

**Coconut sugar** is an all-natural, mild-tasting, and low-glycemic sweetener produced by dehydrating the nectar from coconut buds. It can be used at a 1:1 ratio for regular cane sugar. It can also be used in liquid form as coconut nectar instead of maple syrup.

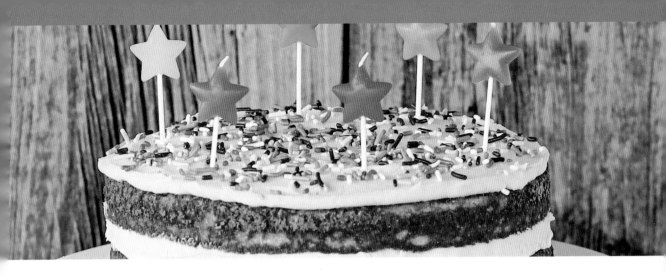

**Honey:** Local raw honey is a delicious and healthy sweetener and most preferred in my home. Raw honey is the sweet liquid that honeybees produce from the concentrated nectar of flowers. Collected straight from the extractor, it is unheated, unpasteurized, and unprocessed.

You can substitute honey for sugar in most baking recipes, but be sure to follow these tips:

- Use ½ to ¾ cup (160 to 240 g) of honey for each 1 cup (200 g) of sugar in the recipe.
- Reduce the liquid by ¼ cup (60 ml) for each 1 cup (200 g) of sugar replaced.
- Reduce the baking temperature by 25°F (10°C) because honey will make your baked goods brown more easily.
- If the recipe doesn't already include baking soda, add ¼ teaspoon for each 1 cup (200 g) of sugar replaced.

Although it's fun to create a unique recipe on occasion, if you're anything like me, you tend to return to a few tried and true standards. For this reason, I chose to incorporate a few grain-free versions of the most familiar and favorite sweet treats: Chocolate Chip Cookies (page 178), Fudgy Brownies (page 177), Banana Nut Bread (page 181), and Dark Chocolate–Dipped Waffle Cones (page 186) will keep your sweet tooth at bay and make it easier to avoid the temptation of their grain-containing counterparts.

And many of these recipes are easily adaptable. Classic Birthday Cake with Buttercream Frosting (page 182) can be made as yellow-vanilla or chocolate, as a double-layered cake, a large sheet cake, or even as cupcakes. Feel free to change up the frosting to suit the occasion—the possibilities are endless!

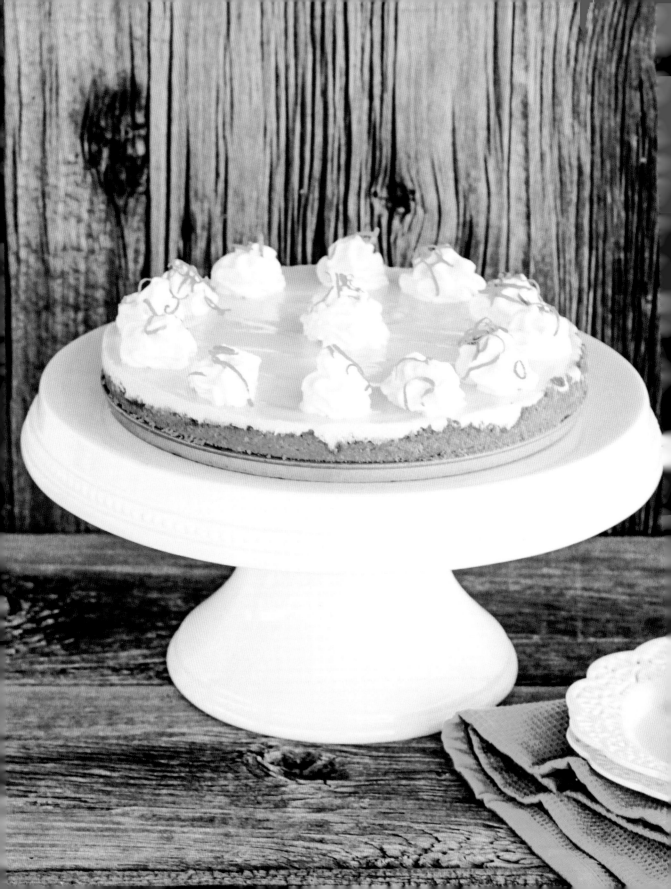

# KEY LIME PIE

I make this fabulously sweet-tart pie for our annual Labor Day Weekend Blue Crab Feast, and it's always a big hit. Although it needs about a day to chill and set, it couldn't be easier to make.

① Preheat the oven to 350°F (180°C, or gas mark 4).

② To make the crust: In a medium bowl, mix together the flours, starch, sugar, butter, gelatin, and salt until it forms a moist, crumbly mixture. Press firmly into a 9-inch (23 cm) pie pan. Bake for 10 minutes. Remove from the oven and allow to cool completely.

③ To make the custard: Using an electric hand mixer, beat the egg yolks in a bowl with the milk and cream until thoapproximately blended. Slowly whisk in the lime juice. Pour the custard into the pie crust and bake for 15 minutes to help the custard begin to set; it will still be slightly jiggly but will finish setting when chilled.

④ Cool the pie on a wire rack until it is at room temperature before covering loosely with plastic wrap and refrigerating overnight.

⑤ Serve with freshly whipped cream, if desired.

## FOR CRUST:

1 cup (112 g) blanched almond flour

1 tablespoon (7 g) coconut flour

¼ cup (32 g) arrowroot starch

¼ cup (48 g) coconut sugar

¼ cup (55 g) butter or ghee, melted

½ teaspoon powdered gelatin

½ teaspoon sea salt

## FOR CUSTARD:

4 large egg yolks

1 can (14 ounces, or 390 g) sweetened condensed milk

¾ cup (175 ml) cold heavy cream

½ cup (120 ml) Key lime juice (fresh squeezed or bottled)

Optional: whipped cream, for serving

YIELD: ONE 9-INCH (23 CM) PIE

**FOR CARROT CAKE:**

2½ cups (280 g) blanched almond flour

¼ cup (28 g) coconut flour

1 tablespoon (7 g) ground cinnamon

1 teaspoon baking soda

½ teaspoon sea salt

½ teaspoon ginger

½ teaspoon nutmeg

⅔ cup (150 g) butter

⅔ cup (213 g) honey

4 large eggs

2 teaspoons vanilla extract

2 cups (220 g) grated carrot

**FOR MAPLE CREAM CHEESE FROSTING:**

16 ounces (455 g) cream cheese, softened

1½ cups (337 g) butter, softened

⅔ cup (160 ml) pure maple syrup

Optional: 1 cup (120 g) chopped walnuts

YIELD: ONE 9 X 13-INCH (23 X 33 CM) CAKE

# CARROT CAKE WITH MAPLE CREAM CHEESE FROSTING

Making a scrumptious grain-free carrot cake is super easy with this recipe. It's moist and flavorful, topped with sweet maple cream cheese frosting. It's one of my favorite fall desserts, especially when enjoyed with a cup of hot coffee.

① Preheat the oven to 350°F (180°C, or gas mark 4) and grease a 9 x 13-inch (23 x 33 cm) pan.

② To make the cake: In a medium bowl, combine the flours, cinnamon, baking soda, salt, ginger, and nutmeg. Mix well and set aside.

③ In a large bowl with a hand mixer or in the bowl of a stand mixer, cream together the butter and honey until light and fluffy, about 2 to 3 minutes. Add the eggs and vanilla and mix well.

④ Slowly add the dry ingredients to the wet and mix well; it will be slightly thicker than pancake batter. Once combined, add the carrots and stir to combine. Let the cake batter rest for 5 minutes.

⑤ Spread the batter into the cake pan and bake for 20 to 30 minutes until a toothpick inserted into the center of the cake comes out clean. Remove from the oven and place on a cooling rack to cool completely.

⑥ To make the frosting: In a large bowl, beat together the cream cheese and butter until light and fluffy, 2 to 3 minutes. Add the maple syrup and mix well. Spread the frosting evenly over the cake and top with the chopped nuts, if desired.

# NO-BAKE COOKIES

Who says you need an oven to make cookies? No-bake cookies are a terrific treat not only on sweltering summer days, but any time. Using shredded coconut instead of oatmeal makes them perfectly grain-free.

½ cup (160 g) honey

¼ cup (60 g) coconut oil

¼ cup (20 g) cocoa powder

2 cups (170 g) shredded coconut (unsweetened)

½ cup (130 g) nut butter (almond, cashew, etc.)

1 teaspoon vanilla extract

YIELD: 16 COOKIES

① In a small saucepan, combine the honey, oil, and cocoa powder and bring to a boil. Boil for 2 minutes, stirring, and then remove from the heat.

② Stir the coconut, nut butter, and vanilla into the hot honey mixture until the nut butter melts and the mixture is smooth.

③ Drop about 2 heaping tablespoons (28 g) of the mixture onto a wax paper–lined baking sheet. Repeat with the remaining cookie dough. Set aside to cool until firm, about 20 minutes. Cookies can be stored in the refrigerator, in a sealed container, for up to a week.

NOTE   Store these cookies in the freezer during the summer for a nice, cool treat.

½ of a recipe for Pie Crust (page 33; store the remaining half of the dough according to recipe directions)

1 cup (192 g) plus 6 tablespoons (72 g) cane sugar, divided

¼ cup (32 g) arrowroot starch

¼ teaspoon sea salt

1½ cups (355 ml) water

Zest and juice of 2 lemons

2 tablespoons (28 g) butter

4 large eggs, separated

YIELD: ONE 9-INCH (23 CM) PIE

# LEMON MERINGUE PIE

Fresh lemon juice and lemon zest make this lovely lemon meringue pie filling so tart. And when it's topped with billows of meringue, it's downright dreamy.

①  Preheat the oven to 350°F (180°C, or gas mark 4).

②  Arrange the pie crust in a 9-inch (23 cm) pie plate and bake for 10 minutes or until lightly brown. Remove from the oven and set aside to cool.

③  In a medium saucepan, whisk together 1 cup (192 g) of the sugar, starch, and salt. Whisk in the water, lemon juice, and lemon zest. Cook over medium-high heat, stirring frequently, until the mixture comes to a boil. Stir in the butter until it's melted and combined.

④  Place the egg yolks in a small bowl and gradually whisk in ½ cup (120 ml) of the sugar mixture. Whisk the egg yolk mixture back into the remaining sugar mixture. Bring to a simmer, lowering the heat if necessary, and continue to cook, stirring constantly, until thick, about 2 to 4 minutes. Remove from the heat. Pour the filling into the baked pastry shell (the filling can be strained if there are lumps).

⑤  In a large glass or metal bowl, whip the egg whites until foamy. Gradually add the remaining 6 tablespoons (72 g) sugar and continue to whip until stiff peaks form, about 3 to 5 minutes. Spread the meringue over the pie, sealing the edges at the crust.

⑥  Bake for 10 minutes or until the meringue is golden brown. Allow to cool before serving.

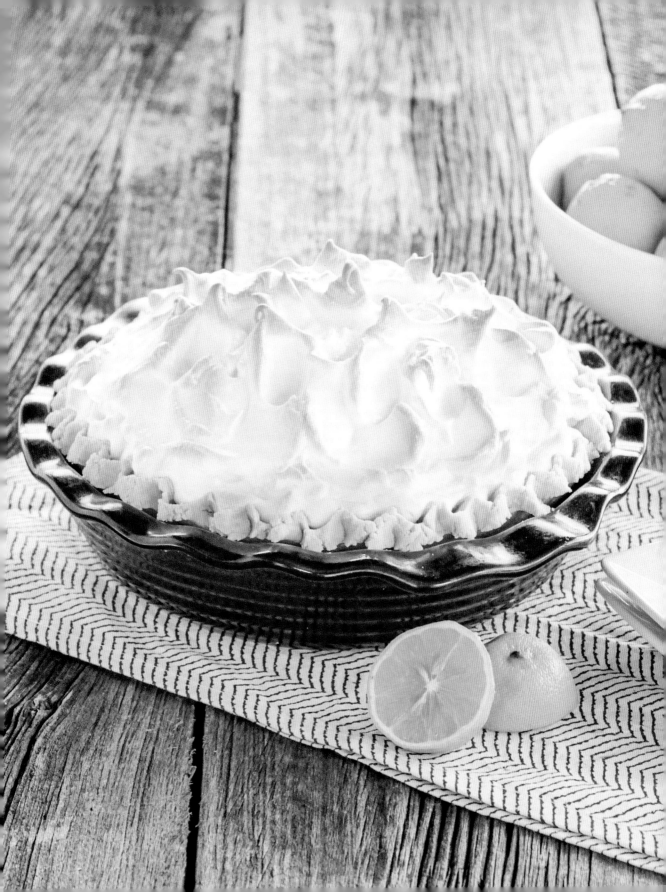

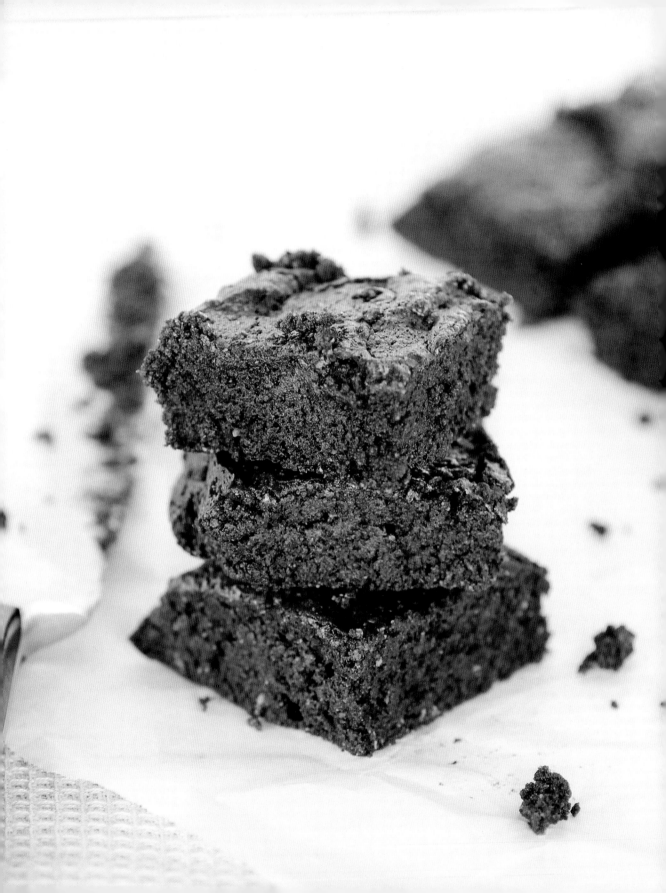

# FUDGY BROWNIES

A chewy, fudgy brownie that is easy to make, these are perfect for a picnic or to just have hanging around for a snack. To transform them into an elegant dessert, top with vanilla ice cream and sliced strawberries.

1 cup (175 g) semisweet or dark chocolate chips

¼ cup (55 g) butter, softened

¾ cup (144 g) coconut sugar

1 teaspoon vanilla extract

½ teaspoon sea salt

2 large eggs, beaten

⅔ cup (75 g) blanched almond flour

⅓ cup (40 g) tapioca starch

Optional: ½ cup (60 g) chopped walnuts

YIELD: 16 BROWNIES

① Preheat the oven to 325°F (170°C, or gas mark 3) and line an 8 x 8 x 2-inch (20 x 20 x 5 cm) baking pan with parchment paper, allowing some of the sides to overhang.

② In the top of a double boiler, melt the chocolate chips and butter, stirring until smooth, and then remove from the heat. Stir in the sugar, vanilla, and salt and allow to cool slightly. Add the eggs and mix throughly.

③ Fold in the almond flour and tapioca starch, stirring until well combined. Add the walnuts, if desired.

④ Pour the brownie batter into the prepared baking pan. Bake for 20 to 25 minutes or until a toothpick inserted into the center comes out clean.

⑤ Remove from the oven and allow to cool for at least 30 minutes. Then gently lift the brownies out with the parchment paper and cut into 16 squares.

NOTE Brownies can be stored in an airtight container at room temperature for up to a week.

1½ cups (168 g) blanched almond flour

½ cup (60 g) tapioca starch

½ teaspoon baking soda

½ teaspoon sea salt

¼ cup (55 g) butter, softened

⅓ cup (64 g) coconut sugar

2 teaspoons vanilla extract

1 large egg

¾ cup (131 g) chocolate chips

Optional: ½ cup (60 g) chopped walnuts or (55 g) pecans

## YIELD: 1 DOZEN COOKIES

# CHOCOLATE CHIP COOKIES

Chocolate chip cookies are a go-to favorite dessert, sweet snack, or after-school treat. With crispy edges and chewy middles, no one will guess these are made healthier, with all real-food ingredients and no grains. In the summer, I like to use these chocolate chip cookies to make s'mores instead of graham crackers and chocolate.

① Preheat the oven to 350°F (180°C, or gas mark 4) and line a cookie sheet with parchment paper.

② In a medium bowl, combine the flour, starch, baking soda, and salt.

③ In a large bowl with a hand mixer or in the bowl of a stand mixer, beat the butter until fluffy, about 2 to 3 minutes. Add the sugar and vanilla and mix well. Beat in the egg until well incorporated. Gradually add the dry ingredients to the wet mixture and mix until smooth with no lumps. Fold in the chocolate chips and nuts, if using.

④ Scoop approximately 2 tablespoons (28 g) of cookie dough, roll into a ball, and set on the prepared cookie sheet. Flatten slightly. Repeat with the remaining dough, setting them 1 inch (2.5 cm) apart. Bake the cookies until golden brown, about 10 to 15 minutes. Transfer to a cooling rack.

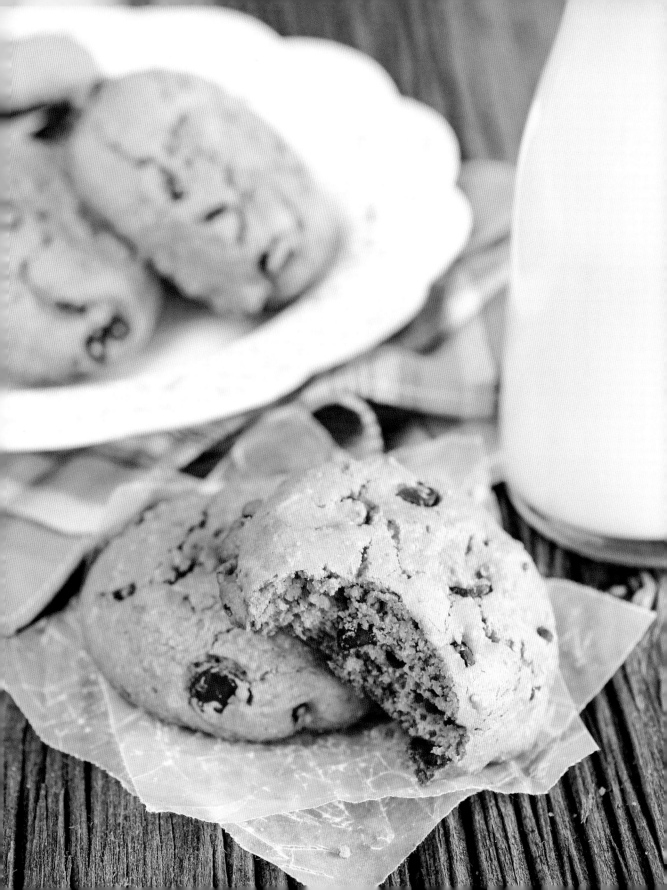

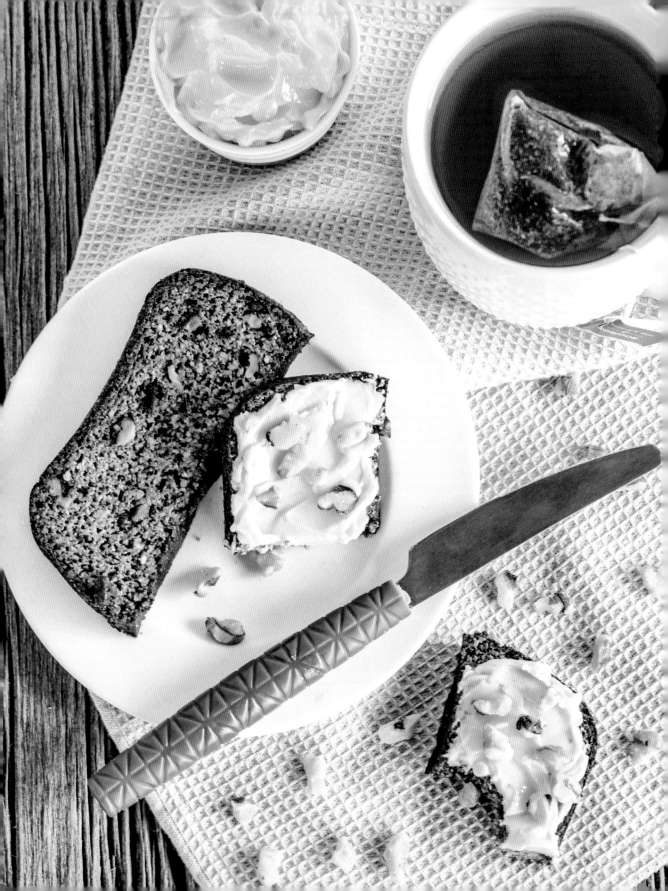

# BANANA NUT BREAD

This banana bread recipe is moist and delicious, with loads of banana flavor. It's wonderful toasted and topped with butter.

① Preheat the oven to 350°F (180°C, or gas mark 4). Grease a 9 x 5 x 3-inch (23 x 15 x 7.5 cm) loaf pan.

② In a food processor, combine the bananas, eggs, maple syrup, water, and vanilla and process until smooth. Add the flour, cinnamon, baking soda, and salt and process until well combined. Pulse in the walnuts, just enough to combine but not chop them up further.

③ Spread the batter in the prepared loaf pan and bake for 45 to 55 minutes until a toothpick inserted into the center comes out clean. Allow to cool in the pan for about 15 minutes and then unmold onto a rack and cool completely before serving.

2 overripe bananas

2 large eggs

¼ cup (60 ml) maple syrup

¼ cup (60 ml) water

¾ teaspoon vanilla extract

2 cups (224 g) blanched almond flour

1 teaspoon ground cinnamon

1 teaspoon baking soda

¼ teaspoon sea salt

⅓ cup (40 g) chopped walnuts

YIELD: ONE 9 x 5-INCH (23 x 15 CM) LOAF

## FOR CAKE:

8 large eggs

1½ cups (355 ml) half-and-half (or ¾ cup [175 ml] milk and ¾ cup [175 ml] heavy cream)

2 teaspoons vanilla extract

1½ cups (288 g) cane sugar

1 cup (112 g) blanched almond flour

1 cup (112 g) coconut flour

1 teaspoon baking soda

½ teaspoon unrefined sea salt

## FOR FROSTING:

½ cup (112 g) butter, softened

3 cups (360 g) powdered sugar

2 tablespoons (28 ml) heavy cream

2 teaspoons vanilla extract

Yield: One 2-layer cake or 20 cupcakes

# CLASSIC BIRTHDAY CAKE WITH BUTTERCREAM FROSTING

This is my favorite recipe in this entire book. Everyone I've ever made it for agrees: it's not just a good grain-free cake, it's one of the best cakes they've ever had.

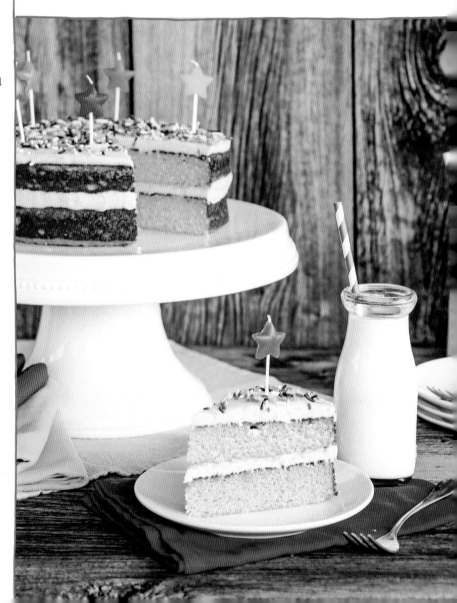

① Preheat the oven to 350°F (180°C, or gas mark 4) and grease two 8-inch (20 cm) cake pans, with a round of parchment paper fitted into the bottom.

② To make the cake: In a large bowl, lightly beat the eggs and then whisk in the half-and-half, vanilla, and sugar.

③ In a smaller bowl, combine the almond flour, coconut flour, baking soda, and salt. Add the dry ingredients to the wet and blend with a handheld mixer.

④ Pour half of the batter into each of the prepared cake pans and bake for 30 minutes or until a toothpick inserted into the center comes out clean.

⑤ Cool for 1 hour in the pan and then remove from the pans and place on a cooling rack to cool completely.

⑥ To make the frosting: In a large bowl with an electric mixer or in the bowl of a stand mixer, beat the butter on high speed until light and fluffy, about 2 to 3 minutes. Add the powdered sugar, ½ cup (60 g) at a time, until completely incorporated and smooth. Mix in the heavy cream and vanilla.

⑦ If the tops of your cakes are uneven or rounded, use a serrated knife to trim to create a flat surface. Place 1 cake on a plate or cake stand, then spread evenly with half of the frosting. Place the other cake on top of the first layer. Spread the remaining frosting on top of the second layer.

⑧ *Chocolate Cake Variation:* Add ½ cup (40 g) cocoa powder, ½ teaspoon baking soda, and an additional ¼ cup (48 g) cane sugar to the dry ingredients.

⑨ *Chocolate Frosting Variation:* Add 2 tablespoons (10 g) cocoa powder before adding the powdered sugar.

NOTES   The frosting recipe is enough to frost a cake as shown in the picture or to frost 20 cupcakes. For more frosting, double the recipe. The cake can be stored in a covered container for up to a week at room temperature.

½ cup (96 g) potato starch

¼ cup (28 g) blanched almond flour

½ teaspoon ground cinnamon

⅓ cup (75 g) butter, softened

¾ cup (144 g) coconut sugar

½ cup (55 g) chopped pecans or (60 g) walnuts

4 cups (440 g) peeled, cored, and thinly sliced apples (4 to 6 apples)

Optional: vanilla ice cream

YIELD: 6 TO 8 SERVINGS

# APPLE CRISP

Although apple crisp doesn't have a crust, there are typically oats and flour in the crumb topping. With just a few simple swaps, you can enjoy apple crisp while eating grain-free. Make sure you have vanilla ice cream on hand to serve this crisp à la mode.

① Preheat the oven to 375°F (190°C, or gas mark 5) and grease an 8 x 8-inch (20 x 20 cm) baking pan.

② In a small bowl, combine the starch, flour, and cinnamon. Using 2 forks or a pastry blender, cut in the butter until it becomes coarse meal. Add the sugar and nuts and mix well.

③ Layer the apple slices in the pan and evenly sprinkle the dry mixture on top.

④ Bake for 30 minutes until brown and crispy on top. Remove from the oven and allow to cool slightly.

⑤ Serve warm with a scoop of ice cream, if desired.

# FUNNEL CAKES

Yes, this is the county fair–type funnel cakes—made grain-free! Light and fluffy, they're served hot, dusted with powdered sugar.

Lard or palm oil, for frying

1 cup (112 g) blanched almond flour

½ cup (60 g) tapioca starch

¼ cup (48 g) coconut sugar

2 teaspoons baking powder (page 20)

1 teaspoon vanilla extract

½ teaspoon sea salt

Powdered sugar, for dusting

### YIELD: 4 TO 6 FUNNEL CAKES

① In a deep skillet or a heavy-bottomed pot, heat 1 inch (2.5 cm) of fat to 325°F (170°C).

② In a blender, combine the flour, starch, sugar, baking powder, vanilla, and salt and blend on high until smooth, about 30 seconds. Pour the mixture into a recycled plastic squeeze bottle or a piping bag.

③ Squeeze a thin stream of batter in a spiderweb shape into the hot oil. Make the funnel cake about 5 inches (12.5 cm) wide (any larger will be very difficult to flip).

④ Fry for 3 to 4 minutes or until golden brown and firm enough to flip. Carefully turn over using a slotted metal spatula and fry for an additional 3 to 4 minutes or until golden brown.

⑤ Remove from the oil and drain on a paper towel–lined plate. Dust with powdered sugar. Funnel cakes are best served fresh.

NOTE   The batter can be stored in the refrigerator and used over several days to make funnel cakes for dessert.

2 large eggs, beaten

⅔ cup (128 g) coconut sugar

⅓ cup (37 g) blanched almond flour

⅓ cup (43 g) arrowroot starch

⅓ cup (40 g) tapioca starch

2 tablespoons (28 g) butter or coconut oil

1 teaspoon vanilla extract

¼ teaspoon sea salt

1 cup (175 g) dark chocolate chips

YIELD: 6 TO 8 WAFFLE CONES

# DARK CHOCOLATE–DIPPED WAFFLE CONES

This recipe requires a waffle cone maker or pizzelle iron and a waffle cone form, because they both make a very thin and crispy waffle. Once you feel comfortable making waffle cones, try filling the cone with ice cream and serving while the cone is still hot.

(1) Preheat a waffle cone maker to medium heat.

(2) In a blender, combine the eggs, sugar, flour, starches, butter, vanilla, and salt and blend on high until smooth, about 30 seconds.

(3) Fill a ¼-cup (60 ml) dry measuring cup with batter and pour into the center of the waffle cone maker (don't scrape out the extra batter from the cup, just keep refilling and pouring until the end and then scrape). Cook for 1 minute and then check for a light brown color; cook for an additional 20 to 40 seconds, if necessary, and/or adjust the setting according to the manufacturer's instructions if the cones are getting too dark or not cooking fast enough.

(4) Quickly remove the waffle cone from the maker and place on a clean dish towel. Use the cloth to help lift and roll the waffle cone around the cone form. Hold the cone for a few seconds to cool into shape and then transfer to a cone holder or set in a tall glass to cool completely. Repeat until all the batter is used.

(5) Melt the chocolate chips in the top of a double boiler. Dip the top of the cones into the melted chocolate. Place the cones back in the cone holder or glasses to allow the chocolate to cool and harden.

(6) Waffle cones will keep in an airtight container for up to a week. Fill with ice cream of your choice and enjoy!

# NO-OATMEAL CREAM PIES

These no-oatmeal cookies, baked just until set, are soft and tender. You can also use the cream filling to frost the Classic Birthday Cake or cupcakes (page 182).

**FOR COOKIES:**

2 cups (224 g) blanched almond flour

¾ cup (90 g) tapioca starch

¼ cup (32 g) arrowroot starch

½ teaspoon ground cinnamon

½ teaspoon sea salt

1 cup (192 g) coconut sugar

⅓ cup (80 ml) milk

3 tablespoons (42 g) butter, melted

2 tablespoons (40 g) honey

1 teaspoon vanilla extract

**FOR FILLING:**

8 ounces (225 g) cream cheese, softened

¾ cup (165 g) butter, softened

⅓ cup (107 g) honey

1 teaspoon vanilla extract

**YIELD: 24 CREAM PIE SANDWICHES**

① Preheat the oven to 325°F (170°C, or gas mark 3) and line a baking sheet with parchment paper.

② To make the cookies: In a medium bowl, whisk together the flour, starches, cinnamon, and salt.

③ In a large bowl with a handheld mixer or in the bowl of a stand mixer on medium speed, beat together the sugar, milk, butter, honey, and vanilla until combined and smooth. Gradually add the dry mixture and mix until combined.

④ Scoop 1-ounce (28 g) portions of dough and arrange 2 inches (5 cm) apart on the baking sheet. Using moistened fingers, flatten each into a ½-inch (1.3 cm)-thick disk. You will need a total of 48 cookies.

⑤ Bake for 18 to 20 minutes or until the cookies spring back when touched. Transfer to a cooling rack. Cool completely.

⑥ To make the filling: In a medium bowl with a handheld mixer or in the bowl of a stand mixer, beat together the cream cheese and butter on high until light and fluffy, about 3 minutes. Add the honey and vanilla and mix until incorporated.

⑦ Turn over half of the cooled cookies. Spread the filling on the flat side and sandwich with another cookie, flat-side against the filling. Repeat for the remaining cookies. Store the cream pies in an airtight container in the fridge for up to a week.

**NOTE** No-Oatmeal Cream Pies can be frozen in an airtight container for up to 6 months. Allow to thaw in the refrigerator overnight before eating.

## FOR CAKE:

- ¼ cup (28 g) blanched almond flour
- ¼ cup (30 g) tapioca starch
- ¼ cup (32 g) arrowroot starch
- ½ teaspoon baking soda
- ½ teaspoon baking powder (page 20)
- ½ teaspoon ground cinnamon
- ½ teaspoon ground cloves
- ¼ teaspoon sea salt
- 3 large eggs
- 1 cup (192 g) coconut sugar
- ⅔ cup (163 g) pumpkin puree
- Optional: 1 cup chopped nuts, such as (120 g) walnuts or (110 g) pecans
- Powdered sugar, for dusting

## FOR FILLING:

- 8 ounces (225 g) cream cheese, softened
- ½ cup (112 g) butter, softened
- 2 tablespoons (40 g) honey
- 2 tablespoons (30 ml) maple syrup
- 1 teaspoon vanilla extract

Yield: 10 servings

# PUMPKIN ROLL WITH CREAM CHEESE FILLING

If you're unfamiliar with pumpkin rolls, then you're in for a real treat. This is a thin pumpkin cake, rolled around a cream cheese filling. It's as pretty as it is delicious. I make several of them before Thanksgiving and keep them in the freezer. Although they are best when thawed in the refrigerator, they are also very good frozen.

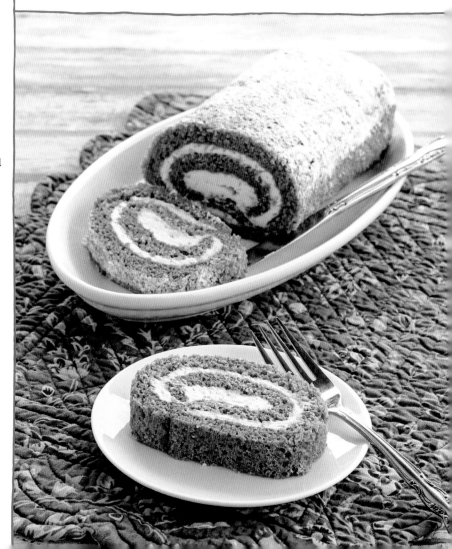

① Preheat the oven to 375°F (190°C, or gas mark 5). Line a 15 x 10-inch (38 x 25.4 cm) jelly-roll pan with lightly greased parchment paper.

② To make the cake: In a medium bowl, combine the flour, starches, baking soda, baking powder, cinnamon, cloves, and salt and mix well.

③ In a large bowl with a handheld mixer or in the bowl of a stand mixer on medium speed, beat together the eggs and coconut sugar until thick. Add the pumpkin puree and blend until combined. Gradually add the dry ingredients and mix until smooth.

④ Pour the batter onto the prepared jelly-roll pan and sprinkle with the chopped nuts, if desired. Bake for 10 to 15 minutes until the top of the cake springs back when touched.

⑤ While the cake is baking, spread out a clean kitchen towel and sprinkle with powdered sugar. When the cake is done, remove it from the oven and gently flip the cake onto the powdered sugared towel, so the parchment paper is on top, and peel off the paper.

⑥ Starting at a short end, roll up the towel and cake together into a jelly roll. Set seam-side down and allow to completely cool while rolled up, about 1 hour.

⑦ To make the filling: In a bowl with a handheld mixer or in the bowl of a stand mixer on medium speed, beat together the cream cheese and butter until fluffy, about 2 to 3 minutes. Add the honey, maple syrup, and vanilla and beat until smooth.

⑧ When the cake is completely cool, gently unroll it and spread with the cream cheese filling to the edges. Roll it back up (without the towel) and wrap in plastic wrap. Chill in the fridge for at least 1 hour before cutting and serving. Dust with powdered sugar, if desired.

NOTE  Pumpkin rolls freeze well, wrapped tightly in plastic wrap, for up to 6 months. (Freeze it in slices so you can take out just what you need.) Allow to thaw overnight in the fridge before serving.

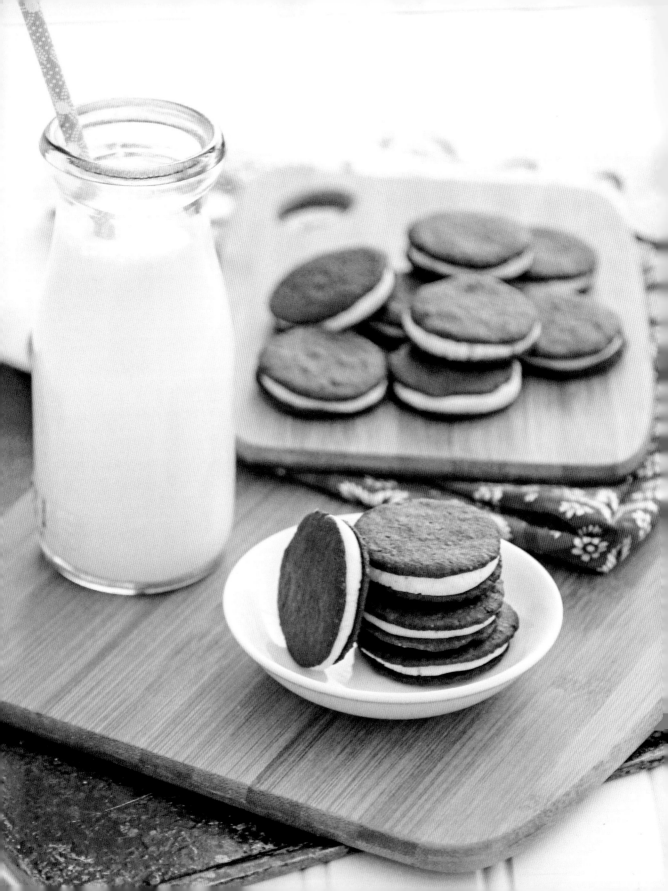

# CHOCOLATE SANDWICH COOKIES

Here's a simple homemade version of your favorite cream-filled chocolate cookie, suitable for dunking into milk. Add a couple drops of peppermint extract to the filling or cookie dough for a chocolate-mint version.

---

① Preheat the oven to 325°F (170°C, or gas mark 3) and line a baking sheet with parchment paper.

② To make the cookies: In a small bowl, whisk together the flour, starches, cocoa powder, potato flour, and salt.

③ In a large bowl with a handheld mixer or in the bowl of a stand mixer on medium speed, beat together the egg, butter, sugar, and vanilla for 1 minute until smooth. Gradually add the flour mixture and beat until well blended, scraping down the sides of the bowl as necessary.

④ Using your hands, roll a teaspoon of dough into a ball and place it on the baking sheet. Use your fingers, lightly dusted with cocoa powder, to press the ball flat into a ¼-inch (6 mm)-thick disk. Repeat for all the dough, placing the cookies 1 inch (2.5 cm) apart from each other. You will need a total of 48 cookies.

⑤ Bake for 9 to 11 minutes or until the cookies look dry. Cool for 5 minutes and then remove from the baking sheet and place on a cooling rack to cool completely before filling.

⑥ To make the filling: Using an electric mixer, beat together the sugar, shortening, and vanilla until well combined. Spread the filling on the flat side of a cookie and top with another cookie. Cookies can be stored in an airtight container at room temperature for up to a week.

## FOR COOKIES:

⅓ cup (37 g) plus 1 tablespoon (7 g) blanched almond flour

⅓ cup (43 g) plus 1 tablespoon (11 g) arrowroot starch

⅓ cup (40 g) plus 1 tablespoon (8 g) tapioca starch

3 tablespoons (15 g) cocoa powder, plus more for dusting

1 tablespoon (11 g) potato flour

¼ teaspoon sea salt

1 large egg

½ cup (112 g) butter, softened

½ cup (96 g) cane sugar

1 teaspoon vanilla extract

## FOR FILLING:

¾ cup (90 g) powdered sugar

½ cup (112 g) palm shortening

1 teaspoon vanilla extract

YIELD: 24 COOKIE SANDWICHES

# CHOCOLATE WHOOPIE PIES

The whoopie pie, or gob (a term indigenous to the Pittsburgh region), is a baked good that may be considered a cookie, a pie, or a cake. It is made of two round mound-shaped pieces of chocolate cake with a sweet, creamy filling or frosting sandwiched between them.

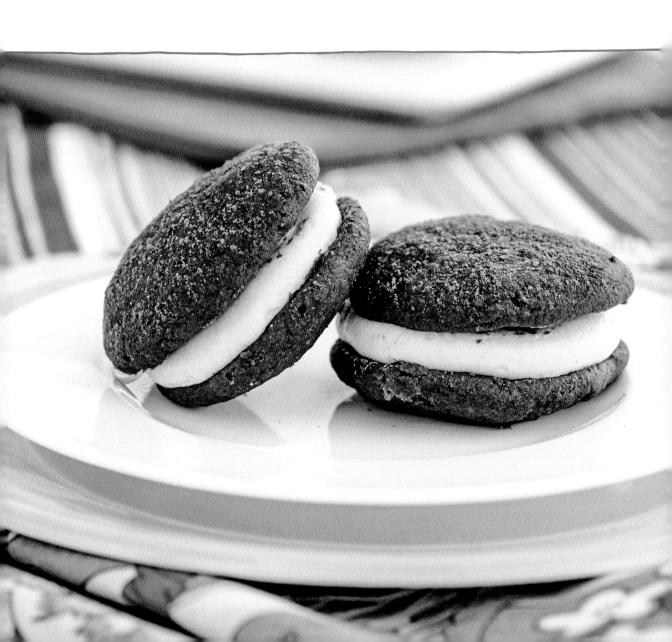

① Preheat the oven to 350°F (180°C, or gas mark 4). Line a baking sheet with parchment paper.

② To make the cakes: In a large bowl with a handheld mixer or in the bowl of a stand mixer on medium speed, beat together the sugar and butter until light and fluffy, about 3 minutes. Add the egg and vanilla and beat until well combined.

③ In a separate bowl, combine the flour, starches, cocoa powder, baking soda, baking powder, and salt. Add half of the dry ingredients to the butter mixture on low speed.

④ When the dry ingredients have been incorporated, stop the mixer and add the buttermilk. Continue to mix on low speed until all the ingredients are incorporated. Add the remaining dry mixture and mix on low until combined.

⑤ Drop heaping tablespoons (15 g) of batter onto the baking sheet, 2 inches (5 cm) apart. Bake for 8 to 10 minutes until the tops of the cakes spring back when touched. Remove from the oven and allow the cakes to cool for 10 minutes before removing from the pan. Cool completely on a cooling rack prior to filling.

⑥ To make the filling: In a large bowl, beat the butter on high until light and fluffy, about 2 to 3 minutes. Add the powdered sugar, ½ cup (60 g) at a time, until completely incorporated. Mix in the heavy cream and vanilla until smooth.

⑦ Spread the filling on the flat side of one cake and sandwich with the flat side of another cake. Whoopie pies can be stored at room temperature in an airtight container for 3 to 5 days.

**FOR CAKES:**

1 cup (192 g) coconut sugar

½ cup (112 g) butter, softened

1 large egg

1 teaspoon vanilla extract

⅔ cup (75 g) blanched almond flour

1 tablespoon (11 g) potato flour

⅔ cup (85 g) arrowroot starch

⅔ cup (80 g) tapioca starch

⅓ cup (27 g) cocoa powder

1 teaspoon baking soda

1 teaspoon baking powder (page 20)

½ teaspoon sea salt

1 cup (235 ml) cultured buttermilk

**FOR FILLING:**

½ cup (112 g) butter, softened

3 cups (360 g) powdered sugar

2 tablespoons (28 ml) heavy cream

1 teaspoon vanilla extract

YIELD: 12 WHOOPIE PIES

## FOR CUPCAKES:

¼ cup (55 g) butter, softened

¼ cup (80 g) honey

½ teaspoon vanilla extract

4 large eggs

¼ cup (28 g) coconut flour

2 teaspoons beet powder

½ teaspoon cocoa powder

¼ teaspoon sea salt

¼ teaspoon baking soda

## FOR FROSTING:

8 ounces (225 g) cream
   cheese, softened

2 tablespoons (28 g) butter,
   softened

2 tablespoons (30 ml) maple
   syrup

YIELD: 8 CUPCAKES

NOTE  Beet powder can be
found at local food co-ops that
have bulk spices or online.

# RED VELVET CUPCAKES WITH CREAM CHEESE FROSTING

Although red velvet cake is a Southern classic, it's traditionally made with unhealthy ingredients such as white flour and red food coloring. Getting its red hue from beet powder, this smooth, moist version has just as much delicious cocoa flavor, making it perfect for Valentine's Day—or any day.

① Preheat the oven to 350°F (180°C, or gas mark 4) and line 8 cups of a cupcake pan with paper liners.

② To make the cupcakes: In a medium bowl with a handheld mixer or in the bowl of a stand mixer on medium speed, beat together the butter, honey, and vanilla until fluffy, about 3 minutes. Add the eggs, one at a time, beating each until well incorporated.

③ Add the flour, powders, salt, and baking soda and mix well. Allow the batter to rest for 15 minutes.

④ Pour the batter into the cupcake cups (about two-thirds full) and bake for 15 to 20 minutes until a toothpick inserted into the center of a cupcake comes out clean.

⑤ Transfer the cupcakes to a cooling rack and allow to cool completely before frosting.

⑥ To make the frosting: In a medium bowl, beat together the cream cheese and butter until light and fluffy, about 2 to 3 minutes. Add the maple syrup and mix well. Frost the cooled cupcakes. Cupcakes can be stored in an airtight container in the refrigerator for 3 to 5 days.

# Afterword
# THE WITHOUT GRAIN LIFESTYLE

Despite whatever doubts you still may have, let me assure you: if I can live without grain, so can you! I've successfully navigated the grain-free terrain for several years without feeling deprived. The secret is making sure you are always prepared and learning how to replicate the foods you might otherwise miss. I've already shared with you 100 recipes to get your started, along with some tips and tricks to creating grain-free versions of your own favorite recipes. Still, every meal isn't going to be under your control, made in your own kitchen.

The next step is getting prepared for those times in which you are at the mercy of someone else to prepare food for you. Holidays, parties, going out to eat—they are an inevitable part of our lives, but they don't have to be a hindrance to a grain-free lifestyle. With the tips that follow, you'll learn how to have foresight and be prepared to succeed in any situation.

I'll also share easy ways to modify the ingredients in this book (and other recipes) to avoid common allergenic foods, such as dairy and eggs. And at the end, I'll provide you with resources for many of the ingredients I've used throughout this book. I hope you'll see that a grain-free lifestyle can be as simple to follow as one with grain—only you'll feel so much better!

# GRAIN-FREE HOLIDAYS

Holiday celebrations brim with food and fun, but they also create special health and dietary challenges for the millions of people with food allergies, intolerances, or diet-controlled diseases. Fortunately, you can still enjoy holiday breads, cookies, pies, and other treats—it just takes planning and creativity. Here are some tips to help you have a holiday season without grain.

**Do your homework.** Knowing which foods you can and cannot eat is crucial. Although breads and pasta dishes are obvious no-no's, learn what other foods—such as casseroles, gravies, salad dressings, and marinades—might also contain grains and look for grain-free alternatives and recipes. When it comes to holiday cheer, wine and cocktails made with tequila, rum, and potato vodka are safe bets, but avoid the beer and wine coolers.

**Plan ahead.** If you are attending a party at someone's home and are unsure of the menu, prepare and bring a dish to share that you know you will be able to eat. If the party is at a restaurant or hotel, call the chef or food service manager for information about the menu. Ask whether there is an allergy/gluten-free menu or whether you can request a special meal. You'll have more success if you call several days to a week in advance. The best time to reach a restaurant or caterer is about 2 p.m.—between the lunch and dinner rush. Once you arrive at the party, confirm that your special meal is being prepared and let the kitchen staff know where you are seated.

**Be assertive.** If you get a salad with croutons, don't just pick them off. Send it back and ask for a fresh-made salad. Even small traces of gluten—such as where the croutons came into contact with the vegetables in your salad—will cause cross-contamination. Tell the server or chef that it's important to use extra care in preparing and serving your food.

If you don't trust the chef, restaurant, or party host or hostess to deliver a safe, grain-free meal, eat something at home before the gathering and just have a beverage, fresh fruit, or another safe alternative at the party.

**Be creative.** Experiment with creating your own grain-free versions of your favorite holiday foods. You would be surprised how easy it be to adapt most recipes, once you learn how the grain-free flours work together. (I've shared my basic combination of grain-free flours to replace all-purpose flour on page 198.)

**Change your focus.** Although food takes center stage during the holiday season, don't forget to relish special time with family and friends. Focusing more on people and less on food can make your holiday more meaningful.

# GRAIN-FREE TIPS FOR EATING OUT

Eating out and staying grain-free might seem like a very difficult task, particularly at first. But if you plan ahead, it doesn't have to be a big deal. Of course, you're probably going to cook a lot more and eat more of your meals at home, at least initially, but it is possible to enjoy the occasional treat, such as a night out with friends.

**Do your research before you leave home!**
Don't wait until you get to the restaurant where you may be rushed into a decision. Take a few minutes to look for the restaurant menu online to see what your options are beforehand or, better yet, give them a call and ask whether they have any allergy-free options.

**Tell *everyone* that you have food allergies.**
No, I don't mean tell strangers on the street or patrons at the next table. I always start by notifying the hostess when I arrive that I have food allergies. I ask if they have an allergy-free and/or gluten-free menu. If they do not have a specifically designated menu, then I'll ask if the manager is available to go over the menu with me to determine which dishes are safe for me to eat.

Every person who comes to your table should know you have allergies, whether they are taking your order or serving your drinks. For example, you can find creative ways to work it into the conversation with the bartender: "I have food allergies and I can't have alcohol made from grains. I prefer vodka. Do you have any potato vodka? Or do you have any recommendations?"

**Never downplay the importance of the way you eat.** By telling people that you have food allergies, you will be taken more seriously than if you say you're on a grain-free "diet." There are so many people who don't yet understand the critical role food plays in our daily health and what an impact removing grains from your diet can make.

Using the term "food allergies" also makes people aware right away that you are not only avoiding one food, but several. When asked for specifics, I've found the best way to explain my food allergies is, "I cannot eat wheat, gluten, or any other grains, such as corn, rice, or oatmeal."

**Don't be too embarrassed to ask.** My mom always tells me, "Ask for nothing, get nothing." Although naturally grain-free foods are readily available, in many forms, at practically every restaurant (eggs, meat, fish, vegetables, etc.), there are many ways that grains can hide in plain sight: sauces, seasonings, marinades, and breadings are just some of the things to be cautious about. (Remember the key culprits from page 18.) When in doubt, ask!

Don't be afraid to ask questions about the ingredients in a dish or how it's prepared. "Can I get the grilled [chicken, steak, or fish] without any seasonings or sauces?"

Also don't hesitate to ask for a convenient swap: "May I have an extra serving of vegetables instead of the rice?" The worst they can say is "no."

You may feel like you're being a bother by asking so many questions or requesting substitutions, but remember that part of their job is to be courteous and helpful to you during your dining experience. Don't let your shyness get in the way of your health.

**Always have a backup plan.** When in doubt, have a few go-to safe meal ideas in mind. My always safe meal is a tossed salad (no bread, breadsticks, crackers, or croutons) with an oil-vinegar dressing. Although it's not the kind of meal I get excited about when eating out, it will hold me over until I get home—and someone else takes care of the dishes.

**Tell them, "Thank you!"** If people have gone out of their way to be helpful, go out of your way to tell them thank you and that you sincerely appreciate their help. And it never hurts to put a little extra in the tip. Next time you come back, they will most likely be even more helpful!

## ALLERGY-FREE SUBSTITUTIONS

| ALLERGEN | SUBSTITUTE | NOTES |
|---|---|---|
| All-purpose flour | Almond flour, sesame seed flour, or cashew flour | 1:1 ratio |
| Eggs | Chia "egg": 1 tbsp (12 g) ground chia seeds plus 3 tbsp (45 ml) water = 1 egg. | Let the mixture sit for 5 minutes before using. |
| | Flax "egg": 1 tbsp (7 g) ground flaxseed plus 3 tbsp (45 ml) water = 1 egg. | Let the mixture sit for 5 minutes before using. |
| | Mashed starchy veggies or fruit such as sweet potato, white potato, pumpkin, applesauce, or banana. | ¼ cup (50 g) = 1 egg |
| | Gelatin and water: 1 tbsp (7 g) gelatin plus 1 tbsp (15 ml) cold water plus 2 tbsp (28 ml) hot water = 1 egg. | Beat until frothy. |
| Milk | Nut milks and coconut milk | 1:1 ratio |
| Heavy cream | Coconut cream | 1:1 ratio |
| Half-and-half | Mix together equal parts coconut milk and coconut cream. | |
| Sour cream | 1 cup (235 ml) coconut cream plus 1 teaspoon lemon juice | 1:1 ratio |
| Buttermilk | 1 cup (235 ml) nondairy milk plus 1 teaspoon apple cider vinegar | 1:1 ratio |
| Yogurt | Coconut yogurt | 1:1 ratio |

# RESOURCES

| ITEM | COMPANY NAME | COMPANY WEBSITE |
| --- | --- | --- |
| Apple cider vinegar | Bragg | www.bragg.com |
| Arrowroot starch | Nuts.com | www.nuts.com |
| Blanched almond flour | Honeyville | http://shop.honeyville.com |
| Bone broth | Pacific Foods<br>Bare Bones Broth | www.pacificfoods.com<br>www.barebonebroth.com |
| Butter | Trickling Springs Creamery | www.tricklingspringscreamery.com |
| Butter | Kalona SuperNatural | www.kalonasupernatural.com |
| Buttermilk, cultured | Trickling Springs Creamery | www.tricklingspringscreamery.com |
| Cane sugar | Nuts.com | www.nuts.com |
| Chocolate, soy-free | Tropical Traditions | www.tropicaltraditions.com |
| Coconut aminos | Coconut Secret | www.coconutsecret.com |
| Coconut flour | Tropical Traditions | www.tropicaltraditions.com |
| Coconut milk (additive-free) | Natural Value | www.naturalvalue.com |
| Coconut oil | Tropical Traditions | www.tropicaltraditions.com |
| Coconut sugar | Madhava | www.madhavasweeteners.com |
| Cottage cheese | Kalona SuperNatural | www.kalonasupernatural.com |
| Cream cheese | Organic Valley | www.organicvalley.coop |
| Dried fruit | Nuts.com | www.nuts.com |
| Fish sauce | Red Boat Fish Sauce | www.redboatfishsauce.com |
| Ghee | Pure Indian Foods | www.purindianfoods.com |
| Grass-fed gelatin | Great Lakes Gelatin | www.greatlakesgelatin.com |
| Half-and-half | Trickling Springs Creamery | www.tricklingspringscreamery.com |
| Heavy cream | Trickling Springs Creamery | www.tricklingspringscreamery.com |
| Honey | Tropical Traditions | www.tropicaltraditions.com |
| Honey | The Family Cow | www.yourfamilyfarmer.com |
| Lard | US Wellness Meats | www.grasslandbeef.com |
| Maple syrup | Tropical Traditions | www.tropicaltraditions.com |
| Mayonnaise | Wilderness Family Naturals | www.wildernessfamilynaturals.com |

| ITEM | COMPANY NAME | COMPANY WEBSITE |
| --- | --- | --- |
| Nutritional yeast | KAL | www.amazon.com |
| Nuts | Nuts.com | www.nuts.com |
| Olive oil | Kasandrinos International | www.kasandrinos.com |
| Palm oil | Tropical Traditions | www.tropicaltraditions.com |
| Palm shortening | Tropical Traditions | www.tropicaltraditions.com |
| Pasture-raised meats | US Wellness Meats | www.grasslandbeef.com |
| Potato flour | Nuts.com | www.nuts.com |
| Potato starch | Nuts.com | www.nuts.com |
| Powdered sugar | Wholesome Sweeteners | http://wholesomesweeteners.com |
| Raw cheese | The Family Cow | www.yourfamilyfarmer.com |
| Raw dairy | The Family Cow | www.yourfamilyfarmer.com |
| Sauerkraut, fermented | Tropical Traditions | www.tropicaltraditions.com |
| Schmaltz | US Wellness Meats | www.grasslandbeef.com |
| Sea salt | Real Salt | www.realsalt.com |
| Seafood, wild-caught | Vital Choice | www.vitalchoice.com |
| Shredded coconut | Tropical Traditions | www.tropicaltraditions.com |
| Sour cream | Kalona SuperNatural | www.kalonasupernatural.com |
| Spices | Simply Organic | www.simplyorganic.com |
| Spices, organic | Frontier Co-op | www.frontiercoop.com/products/spices.php |
| Stevia | SweetLeaf | www.sweetleaf.com |
| Tallow | US Wellness Meats | www.grasslandbeef.com |
| Tapioca starch | Nuts.com | www.nuts.com |
| Uncured meats | AppleGate Farms | www.applegate.com |
| Vanilla extract | Tropical Traditions | www.tropicaltraditions.com |
| Worcestershire sauce | Lea and Perrins | www.leaperrins.com |
| Yogurt | Kalona SuperNatural | www.kalonasupernatural.com |

For help finding local farms, visit www.eatwild.com, www.localharvest.org, www.pickyourown.org, and www.buyfreshbuylocal.net.

# ACKNOWLEDGMENTS

To everyone who has visited my *Health Starts in the Kitchen* blog and/or followed me on social media, I am immensely grateful for your continued support. Without all of you, this book would not have been possible.

To my parents: thank you for raising me to be a confident, unique individual, who isn't intimidated by anyone or anything. I love you both very much. Dad, I followed your advice, and I found something I love to do and made it my career.

Thank you to all of my friends and family who taste-tested recipes for this book. I appreciate you going out of your way to stop over and give me feedback on my latest creations.

Grammie Elsie, Nan Ryczek, and Momma Rich: there are no other women more influential in empowering me to go against the grain and be an accomplished domestic woman. Our talks about cooking and gardening made me understand that my true calling in life was not to be confined in an office, but being barefoot in my garden and sharing my love through food. With love and admiration I thank you for all that you taught me and being forever in my heart, cheering me on when faced with hesitation and faltering confidence. Every day I strive to make you proud of the woman I have become.

Thank you to all my farmer friends who continue to amaze me with their dedication to providing a robust harvest of nourishing foods. To The Family Cow, Working H Farms, DeBerry Farm, Evans Knob Farm, Backbone Food Farm, and all the other famers at the Morgantown Farmers Market: I appreciate your friendship and am proud to have used your foods in the recipes and photographs in this book.

A special thank you to my entire team at Fair Winds Press. I appreciate all of your help and support in writing this book, especially Jill Alexander. Jill, thank you for reaching out to me and seeing potential in my voice.

Hercules, you have been the best companion throughout writing this book. Having you by my side, always ready with puppy kisses and snuggles, made even the most hectic days of recipe failures filled with love and happiness.

And last but not least, thank you to my loving and supportive husband, Ray. Thank you for putting up with a messy kitchen and not complaining when I served you dinner that wasn't nearly as pretty as the pictures (and often cold) while writing this book. I'm humbled at how selflessly you support my endeavors and work so hard to give me everything I've ever wanted. I love you.

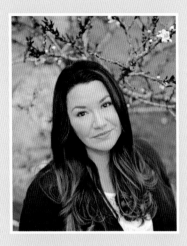

# ABOUT THE AUTHOR

Hayley Barisa Ryczek is the voice behind the healthy cooking and natural lifestyle blog, *Health Starts in the Kitchen*.

Most often you will find Hayley in her kitchen because she has an insatiable passion for food and cooking. She resides with her husband, Ray, and black lab, Hercules, on a 6-acre homestead in rural, southwestern Pennsylvania. Together, they have a beautiful organic garden, raise chickens and turkeys, forage for wild edibles, and enjoy Sunday evening rides in the scenic Laurel Mountains.

# INDEX